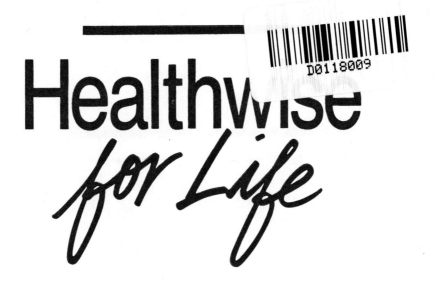

Healthwise for Life

Medical Self-Care for Healthy Aging

Molly Mettler, MSW and Donald W. Kemper, MPH

A Healthwise™ Publication
Healthwise, Inc., Boise, Idaho

Standard Healthwise cover design by Beth Workman

Illustrations by Consuelo Udave

Copyright© 1992 by Healthwise, Incorporated, P.O. Box 1989, Boise, Idaho 83701

First Edition, 1992 (Second Printing, 1992)

ISBN No. 1-877930-02-4

Printed in the United States of America

TABLE OF CONTENTS

PART III: STAYING HEALTHY AND INDEPENDENT

PART IV: Caregiver's Guide

PART V: SELF-CARE RESOURCES

INDEX

To Our Readers

No book can replace the need for doctors--and no doctor can replace the need for people to care for themselves. The purpose of this book is to help you and your doctors work together to manage your health problems.

Healthwise for Life includes basic guidelines on how to recognize and cope with 115 of the most common health problems facing older adults. These guidelines are based on sound medical information provided by physicians, nurses, pharmacists, physical therapists and other health professionals. We have worked to present the information in a straight-forward way that is free from medical jargon. We hope you find it easy to read and easy to use.

This book is as good as we can make it, but we cannot guarantee that it will work for you in every case. Nor will the authors or publishers accept responsibility for any problem that may develop from following its guidelines. Should you receive professional advice that conflicts with the information in the book, look first to your health professional. Because your doctor is able to take your specific medical condition into account, his or her recommendations may prove to be the best. Likewise, should any self-care recommendations fail to provide positive results within a reasonable period, you should consult a health professional.

We are continually adding to and improving this book. If you have a suggestion that will make this book better, please send it to Healthwise for Life Suggestions, c/o Healthwise, P.O. Box 1989, Boise, Idaho, 83701.

We wish you the best of health.

Molly Mettler and Donald W. Kemper

About Healthwise

Healthwise is a nonprofit organization whose mission is "to help people do a better job of staying healthy and taking care of their health problems." Since its founding in 1975, Healthwise has won awards of excellence and recognition from the Centers for Disease Control, the U.S. Department of Health and Human Services, the American Society on Aging and the World Health Organization.

Healthwise works with organizations wishing to enhance the individual's role in health care. Our clients range from volunteer organizations and church groups to Fortune 500 companies, major unions, state governments, hospitals, insurers and HMO's.

Healthwise has published five books, all with workshops and training to support them.

The **Healthwise Handbook** and the Healthwise Workshop. The use of informed medical self-care to improve the quality of care given at home and to help reduce health care costs.

Healthwise for Life and the Healthwise for Life Workshop. Basic medical self-care information, specifically tailored to the health needs of older adults.

Pathways: A Success Guide for a Healthy Life and the Pathways to Health Workshops. A guilt-free approach to health changes in ten areas. The book and workshops are designed to help people make the healthy changes they most want to make.

Growing Wiser: The Older Person's Guide to Mental Wellness and the Growing Wiser Workshops. Memory improvement, mental vitality, coping with loss and life change, maintaining independence and self-esteem for older adults.

The **Growing Younger Handbook** and the Growing Younger Workshops. Fitness, relaxation, nutrition and self-care for older adults aged 60 and better.

In addition to these books and workshops, Healthwise has produced videotapes and other instructional aids to support health promotion efforts. For more information contact Healthwise, P.O.Box 1989, Boise, Idaho, 83701, (208)345-1161 or FAX (208)345-1897.

Acknowledgments

We are particularly grateful to you, the reader. Your interest in actively managing your health problems makes this book possible.

Special thanks also goes to members of the Healthwise staff. Diana Stilwell, MPH, contributed greatly to the book with her comments, reviews, and tireless fact-checking. Gene Drabinski, RN, provided invaluable insights into how people learn about their health and what they need to make better health care decisions. Cindy Krieg was responsible for the design and format as well as making sure the book got to print. Betty Matzek was the keeper of the flame, filing and cataloging the latest in medical information and ensuring that we never forgot who would be reading this book. Cimbria Badenhausen, Cindy Hovland, Sara Lorance and Phyllis Tomlinson helped get the manuscript ready. We thank you all.

This book would not have been possible without the extensive help and guidance we received from the following health professionals. We depend upon them for accurate information, the latest medical developments and spirited debate.

Physicians

Catherine Bannerman, MD

Christopher C. Colenda, III, MD, MPH

Bruce V. Davis, MD

Leonard W. Knapp, MD

Robert B. Monroe, MD

Marijo Perry, MD

Dennis E. Richling, MD

Steven Schneider, MD

Mary Beth Tupper, MD

Lester Breslow, MD, MPH

Ginger Dattilo, MD

Chester Durnas, MD

Steve Monamat, MD

Beverly Parker, MD

James T. Pozniakas, MD

Robert Schmidt, MD, MPH, PhD

David Sobel, MD, MPH

Nurses

Ryu Kanemoto, MN, RNC

Jane Mayfield, RN

Mary Lou Long, RNC, MSN

Health Educators

Bernice Bennett, MPH, CHES

Bob Gorsky, PhD

Diane Katz, MPH

Eileen Mackle-Kern, MHA

Susan Eisendrath, MPH

Joan Greathouse, MEd

Joe Leutzinger, MS

Psychologists

Karen Magee, MA

James Read, PhD

Dentist

Edwin O. Matthes, DDS

Pharmacist

Doris Denney, RPh

Physical Therapist

Lynn Johnson, PT

Nutritionist

Ruth Schneider, RD

Finally, we would like to thank the panel of consumers who helped us make this book easy to understand and easy to use:

Nancy Adrian

Joe Braun

Bonnie Mettler

Marty Shepherd

Chuck Thompson

Grace Tucker

Loyal Barker

Margaret Burris

Pris Pontefract

Mae States

Dee Thompson

Ralph Tucker

Introduction

Healthwise for Life can help you improve your health and lower your health care costs. It is a book you may turn to time and again as health problems arise.

The book is divided into five sections:

Your Role in Health Care. What you need to know in order to be a wise medical consumer.

Self-Care for Health Problems. Prevention, treatment, and when to call a doctor for over 115 common illnesses and injuries.

Staying Healthy and Independent. Tips and techniques for fitness, nutrition, stress management, mental wellness, and staying independent.

Caregiver's Guide. Special advice on how to care for yourself as you care for others.

Self-Care Resources. How to manage medications and what you need to have on hand in your home to cope with health problems.

Most people will not read through the book cover to cover in one sitting; it is more of a topic-by-topic book. Look up what you need when a problem or interest arises. However, we do recommend that you read pages 1 and 2 and three special chapters right away.

Page 1 is the "**Healthwise Approach,**" a process to follow every time a health problems arises.

Page 2, the "**Ask-the-Doctor Checklist,**" will help you get the most out of every doctor visit.

Chapter 1, **The Wise Medical Consumer,** offers important information that you can use to improve the quality and lower the cost of the professional care you need.

Chapter 2, **Prevention and Early Detection,** indicates which routine screening tests make the most sense for those aged 50 and better.

Chapter 26, **Your Home Health Center,** lists medications, supplies, and self-care equipment that you may wish to keep in stock.

The rest of the book is there when you need it. We hope it will help you succeed in better managing your own health problems.

The Healthwise Approach

Step One: Observe the Problem

- Describe the problem (Onset? Symptoms? How steady? How intense?):
  _____

- Other unrelated symptoms: _____

- Changes in your life (stress, medications, food, exercise, etc.): _____
  _____

- Vital signs: Temperature _____   Blood pressure _____/_____

  Pulse _____/minute   Breathing _____/minute

  Other home tests _____

- Have you had this problem before?   _____ No   _____ Yes
  If yes, what did you do? _____
  _____

  Previous visits for this problem?   _____ No   _____ Yes   _____ Last visit?
  Results (drugs, tests, improvements): _____

- What self-care have you done (medications, treatments, etc.)? _____
  _____

Step Two: Learn More About It

- Healthwise for Life (note page numbers): _____
- Other books and articles: _____
- People (lay or professional advice): _____

Step Three: Make an Action Plan

- Your "tentative" diagnosis: _____
- Action and support plan: _____
- When to call your physician: _____

Step Four: Evaluate Your Progress

- Are your actions working? _____
  _____

Ask-The-Doctor Checklist

Before the visit:

- Complete the Healthwise Approach on page 1 (take with you).
- Take a list of medications and record of last visit for similar problem.

During the visit:

- Describe the main problem and symptoms (use page 1).
- Describe past experiences with the same problem.

Write down: Temperature _____   Blood pressure_____/_____

- Other tests: _____
- Doctor's diagnosis: _____
- Probable cause: _____
- Recommendations: _____

For medications, tests and treatments, ask:

- What is its name? _____
- Why it is needed? _____
- Costs and risks? _____
- Are there alternatives? _____
- What if I do nothing? _____
- Effect on other medications? _____
- How do I prepare for the test/treatment? _____
- What else can I do at home? _____
- Danger signs/reasons to call back? _____
- **Other problems to discuss (if there is time)** _____

_____

After the visit (complete with your doctor):

- Am I to return for another visit?   _____ No   _____ Yes
  When? _____Why? _____
- Am I to phone in for test results?   _____ No   _____ Yes   _____When?
- What danger signs should I look for? _____
- Should I report back to the doctor by phone for any reason?
  _____ No   _____ Yes   If yes, when? _____
- What else should I know? _____

_____

Each patient carries his own doctor inside him. We are at our best when the doctor who resides within each patient has the chance to go to work.
Albert Schweitzer, M.D.

1

The Wise Medical Consumer

The quality and the cost of medical care depends more on you than on your doctor.

A wise medical consumer is skilled at buying medical care. By following a few basic principles, you can help your doctor improve the care you receive. And, you can lower your own medical costs.

This chapter will help you become a wise medical consumer.

Medical Consumer Principles

1. Good medical care depends on you.
2. Work in partnership with your doctor.
3. Become skilled at buying medical care.
4. Trust your common sense.

Principle 1: Good Medical Care Depends on You

No matter how good your doctor is, you can do a lot to improve the quality of care that you receive. Your doctor cannot practice good medicine without your help. If you expect too much from your doctor and too little from yourself, you may be limiting the quality of care you receive.

What Kind of Medical Consumer Are You?

The chart on page 5 describes two types of medical consumers: passive patients and active patients.

Passive patients rarely question their doctors. Believing that their health problems are the responsibility of their doctors, passive patients expect their doctors to figure out what is wrong and to tell them what they should do about it.

Consumer Types - continued

Passive patients let the doctor ask the questions and then do what the doctor suggests.

Active patients expect to help make medical decisions. They ask questions and learn as much as they can about their medical problems. Active patients work with their doctors to develop effective treatment plans.

Sharing Decisions with Your Doctor

Being a passive patient is sometimes a good option. The passive patient approach works in emergencies, when split-second decisions are needed. It is also the preferred strategy for people who do not want to think about treatment options. If you prefer being a passive patient, you will usually get high quality care at a reasonable cost **if** you have a primary doctor who has your best interests at heart.

Most people, however, will benefit from sharing treatment decisions. When you and your doctor work together, the result is almost always better than when your doctor works alone. There are two basic reasons for this: you know more about yourself than your doctor knows, and you can concentrate more on yourself than your doctor can.

Who Knows You Best?

Doctors have a tough job. They have to make treatment recommendations for lots of people who they don't know very well. Too often, they have to prescribe a treatment that will work best for the average patient.

However, you may not be an average patient.

The average patient may not be willing to try exercise, diet changes, or stress reduction as a treatment plan. If you are willing to try these methods, you need to tell your doctor.

The average patient may prefer to get a prescription every time he or she visits the doctor. If you don't, you need to speak up.

The average patient may want to get rid of the health problem at all costs. You may want to learn about the side effects of treatment before deciding to accept it.

The average patient may want the doctor to perform as many tests as necessary to be absolutely sure what is wrong. You may wish to avoid tests that will not change the treatment plan.

You alone are qualified to decide what's best for you. Tell your doctor your point of view on each decision.

Who Has the Time to Think About You?

You have only one patient to worry about. Your doctor may have thirty per day.

You have the time to think through your case carefully. Your doctor may be facing a full waiting room.

You can look up your symptoms and carefully consider what might have caused them. Your doctor often has to make a treatment decision on the spot. According to the American Society of Internal Medicine, doctors base 70 percent of all diagnoses on what their patients tell them.

If you do a better job of reporting your symptoms, your doctor can do a better job of discovering what is wrong.

Principle 2: Work in Partnership with Your Doctor

Neither you nor your doctor can do it alone. For the best medical care, you need to work together. Here are eight simple steps that will help you work in partnership with your doctor.

Medical Consumer Models

The Passive Patient

Description

Relies on the doctor's advice. Does not ask many questions or offer much information unless asked.

Message

"I'm looking for a doctor who will take charge of all my health problems. I plan to rely on the doctor's judgment in all medical decisions."

Appropriate Situations

- You have one main doctor that you trust to provide or coordinate all needed care.

- You are in an emergency situation where split-second decisions are critical.

The Active Patient

Description

Actively shares in making treatment decisions with the doctor. Is comfortable asking questions and expressing concerns. Strives for a working partnership with the doctor.

Message

"I'm looking for a doctor who will listen to me and involve me fully in treatment decisions. I will share responsibility for choosing among treatment alternatives."

Appropriate Situations

- You are confident your ideas will improve the quality of care you get. You believe your ideas will help keep costs down.

- You do not have a primary physician who is coordinating all of your care.

---

1. Tell your doctor(s) you want to be a partner in treatment decisions.

Your doctor probably has lots of patients who just want the doctor to tell them what to do. If you say nothing, your doctor may assume that you don't want to be involved either.

Write your doctor a short letter and hand-deliver it at your next appointment. Tell him you would like to work with him to make decisions about tests, referrals, and treatments. Also, indicate that you will want to have a good idea of the costs, benefits, and risks of a treatment or test before going ahead with it.

Before surgery or other major medical procedures, give a letter to your doctor highlighting your concerns and desires regarding treatment. The letter will help you and your doctor develop a mutually agreed-upon plan.

Make it clear that in case of emergencies, you don't want the letter to hinder your doctor from doing what he or she thinks is best. Treat it as a plan--but one that can be altered if problems arise.

2. Be honest with your doctor.

You cannot have an effective partnership with your doctor without being open and honest about your plans. If you don't plan to take a prescribed drug, say so. If you are upset or worried, tell your doctor about your concerns.

3. Prepare for office visits.

Most doctor visits are short. If you are prepared, you get what you need from a short visit. Complete the **Healthwise Approach** on page 1 before the visit and take it with you. It will help you focus your visit time on the main problem. The first few minutes are particularly important. Describe the main problem and symptoms first. Later, if there is time, you can ask about other health concerns.

Complete the **Ask-the-Doctor Checklist** on page 2 while you are with the doctor. It will help you organize your questions and record the doctor's answers.

You may copy pages 1 and 2 for your family's use.

4. Ask "why?"

Always ask "why?" before agreeing to any medical test, medication, or treatment. By asking "why?", you will often discover alternatives that may better meet your needs.

5. Ask about alternatives.

Don't automatically jump at the first treatment proposed. There is always at least one other course of action--to wait. Ask your doctor if watchful waiting is appropriate. If yes, use the waiting period to learn more about alternative treatments.

6. Do your own research.

Don't rely solely on what your physician tells you. Your search may turn up new options that your physician did not yet think of. New information could help him or her improve your treatment plan.

Ask if there is a consumer health information service at your local library or hospital. Bookstores may also have good information that can help. If you can't find what you need locally, Planetree Health Resource Center in San Francisco may be able to help. See Resource B4 on page 349.

7. Write it down.

The faintest ink is more accurate than the strongest memory. During the appointment, keep pen and paper handy. Take notes on all important information. Often, the most valuable part of a doctor visit is the information that your doctor gives you about your particular situation. Writing it down ensures that you will go home with what you paid for.

For even better understanding, take along a friend. A second pair of eyes, ears, and hands can be very helpful in recording the doctor's findings and suggestions.

8. Review and summarize.

At the end of the visit, ask if you can briefly repeat from your notes what you think the doctor said. If the doctor corrects your description, change your notes.

Good written records are also important at home. They can help you learn how to better care for a health problem if it happens again.

For Every Doctor Visit

1. Bring:
   - The **Healthwise Approach** (page 1)
   - The **Ask-the-Doctor Checklist** (page 2)
   - A list of all your medications
2. Be honest with your doctor.
3. Ask "why?"
4. Ask about alternatives.
5. Write down important information.
6. Review and summarize.

Consumer tip: Wear clothes that you can remove easily. The time saved in undressing may allow more time with your doctor.

Choosing the Right Doctor

Everyone needs a regular doctor. A host of specialists working on separate health problems may not look at the whole picture.

Pick one physician as your primary doctor and ask him or her to coordinate all your care.

If you are generally in good health, a family physician or internist is a good choice. These doctors are able to handle a broad range of problems.

A geriatrician is a physician who has received special training in the care of older people. Geriatricians are particularly skilled at helping older

Choosing a Doctor - continued

patients who are dealing with several chronic illnesses.

Consider using a specialist for your primary doctor only if you have a long-term chronic condition that tends to dominate your health.

If you have a good working relationship with a doctor who coordinates your care, great! If you need to find one, here is a good way to go about it.

Step 1: Find a few to choose from.

- Ask your friends who they like. Ask other doctors or nurses. Also, many hospitals have a referral service for their staff physicians.

- The local Medicare office can tell you which physicians, by specialty, accept Medicare assignment (acceptance of the fees that Medicare sets for medical care).

  Look under "Medicare Information" in the community services section of your telephone book.

- Ask your insurer or health plan for a list of physicians eligible for maximum benefits.

Step 2: Talk with the office staff.

Call or visit the receptionist. Tell her that you are looking for a new doctor. Ask these questions and record the answers:

- At which hospitals does the doctor have admitting privileges?

Who Works on What?

Cardiologist (MD): heart

Dermatologist (MD): skin

Endocrinologist (MD): diabetes and glandular problems

Family Practitioner (MD): primary care

Gastroenterologist (MD): digestive system

Geriatrician (MD): older adults

Gynecologist (MD): female reproductive system

Internist (MD): primary care

Neurologist (MD): disorders of the brain and nervous system

Oncologist (MD): cancer

Ophthalmologist (MD): eyes

Optometrist (OD): eye care when disease is not involved

Orthopedist (MD): surgery on bones, joints, muscles, etc.

Podiatrist (DPM): foot care

Psychiatrist (MD): mental and emotional problems

Psychologist (MA or PhD): mental and emotional problems

Pulmonologist (MD): lungs

Rheumatologist (MD): arthritis and rheumatism

Urologist (MD): urinary and male reproductive systems

- What are the office hours?

- If I called right now for a routine visit, how soon could I be seen?

- How much time is allowed for a routine visit?

- Will the doctor discuss health problems over the phone?

- Will the doctor make home visits? What will he do if I am too sick to come to the office?

- Does the doctor accept Medicare assignment? (If not, your medical care may cost you more.)

- Will the office complete insurance forms for me?

- What are the terms of payment? Is there a finance charge if I don't pay all at once? (Also, if you need a particular procedure performed on a regular basis, ask what that procedure would cost.)

If you like the answers you get and the "feel" of the office, ask the receptionist if you can briefly meet with the doctor for no charge. If you can, schedule a meeting. If not, ask to schedule a telephone appointment.

Step 3: Talk with the doctor.
This step is important even if you have already decided to choose the doctor.

- Tell the doctor that you are looking for a physician who will listen to your concerns.

- Tell the doctor that you would like to share in making treatment decisions. Ask if he or she will support that. Also ask if your medical records will be available to you if you ask to see them.

- Ask the doctor what is expected of patients.

- Ask how patients your age are treated differently from younger patients. (You want someone who understands that older adults have special medical needs--not someone who attributes all problems to "old age.")

Doctors to Avoid

Most doctors are honest, dedicated professionals. Unfortunately, a few doctors are not.

- Does the doctor suggest anything that seems unethical or illegal?

- Does the doctor prescribe medicines or give injections on every visit?

- Does the doctor promise too much? Beware of any doctor who promises a no-risk cure.

The best way to protect yourself is to ask questions and be observant. If you don't like what you see, find another doctor.

Choosing a Doctor - continued

By asking questions like these, you can determine if you and the physician can work as partners in your health care.

Principle 3: Become Skilled at Buying Medical Care

The best way to buy good medical care is to find a good doctor and to become actively involved in sharing treatment decisions. In addition, you can develop skills to help you avoid unnecessary tests, medications, emergency services, and surgeries that are not in your best interests.

Get More Out of Fewer Medical Tests

Generally, we tend to think that the more information we have on our health, the better. A wise consumer knows that medical tests sometimes do more harm than good.

Medical tests can cause four types of problems:

- False positive results. If the test says you have a problem when you don't, it may lead to inappropriate and expensive testing and treatments.

- False negative results. If you have a problem that the test does not catch, you may miss the opportunity for appropriate treatment.

- Test-caused health problems. Many medical tests carry some risk of causing other problems; for some tests the risks are high. Always ask about problems associated with the test.

- Unneeded expense and pain. If the test results are not likely to change your treatment plan, the cost, inconvenience, and discomfort of the test may not be worth the information.

Medical Test Questions

Before you agree to any medical test, ask these questions:

- Why is the test needed? How will the results change the treatment?

- Is the test accurate and definitive?

  ○ How often will it say that something is wrong when there is not (false positive)?

  ○ How often will it say I'm healthy when I'm not (false negative)?

- What are the risks involved? Are there less risky tests to determine the same thing?

- What are the costs in money, time, and discomfort?

- What are the consequences if I delay or avoid this test?

If a test seems costly, risky, and not likely to change the recommended treatment, ask your doctor if you can avoid it. Try to come to an agreement with your doctor about the best approach. **No test can be done without your permission.**

Increase the Accuracy of the Test

Once you have agreed to medical testing, ask what you can do to reduce the chance of error. Should you restrict food, exercise, alcohol, or medications before the test?

Delays in processing a specimen can cause inaccurate results. Temperatures that are too high or too low can also reduce test accuracy. Ask how your specimen will be handled. If you have reason to doubt the accuracy of a test, ask your physician for another test.

Test Results

Always ask the doctor to show you the full results when they come back. If you can't make a copy, take notes so that you can record the outcome in your home medical records.

If you get an abnormal and unexpected test result, don't automatically believe it. Because medical tests are often inaccurate, it's smart to repeat the test or look for other ways to confirm the diagnosis before agreeing to treatment plans.

Which Drugs to Say "Yes" To

The best way to avoid medications is to stop expecting them. Some people anticipate leaving every doctor visit with a prescription. That assumption sometimes results in the doctor prescribing something that is not necessary. Instead, be reluctant to accept a medication until you know more about it.

Before you agree to take any medication, ask:

- Why do I need it and how does it work?

- What will happen if I choose not to take it?

- When and how should this medication be taken?

- What are its possible side effects?

- What will it cost? Is there a less expensive "generic equivalent" available?

- How will this drug affect the other drugs I take? (Show the doctor a list of all prescription and non-prescription drugs you take.)

Once you and your doctor have agreed on a medication, use good consumer skills to buy it. Medications needed daily for a long period of time can be purchased for less through mail-order companies. However, at times it is more important to have the help of a local pharmacist.

Another option to reduce medication costs is generic equivalents to name-brand drugs. With few exceptions, generic equivalents are just as good and can be purchased for less.

More information on how to manage medications is included in Chapter 25, beginning on page 327.

Wise Use of Emergency Services

In life-threatening situations, modern emergency services are worth their weight in gold. However, for routine services they often cost far more than they are worth. Use good judgment in choosing when to use emergency medical services.

Hospital emergency rooms are set up to handle trauma and life-threatening crises. They are not set up to care for routine illnesses, nor do they follow a first-come, first-served procedure.

During busy times, people with minor illnesses may wait for hours.

Routine services cost much more in emergency departments. There is usually a minimum fee. Also, your records are not available. Emergency room doctors have little information on your medical history.

When you do need to seek care in an emergency department, try to get the most from it. Call your doctor first. If needed, your physician can meet you there. Also review pages 1 and 2 of this book; asking questions of

---

Using an Ambulance

Reasons to Call an Ambulance

- There is an emergency. You need help.

- You are alone with a person who needs immediate care.

- The person has heart attack symptoms: severe chest pain, sweating, shortness of breath. See page 84.

- There is severe bleeding. Apply pressure on the wound while someone else calls for an ambulance.

- You suspect a spinal or neck injury.

Reasons NOT to Call an Ambulance

- There is no emergency.

- The person is conscious and acting normally.

- Anxiety. An unnecessary ambulance ride can add to the person's anxiety about the situation.

- Cost. Emergency medical services are expensive. Most insurers pay for such services only if the problem can be shown to be a true emergency.

- Consideration. Emergency services are best saved for victims of true emergencies.

emergency room professionals is particularly important because they do not know you, nor do they have access to your medical records.

Prepare for the Emergency Room
If there is time, take this book and your medical records with you.

- Use page 1, the **Healthwise Approach**, to help you think through the problem and report symptoms to the doctor.

- Use page 2, the **Ask-The-Doctor Checklist**, to organize questions for the doctor.

- See page 10 to review the medical test checklist.

- Use your home medical records to discuss your medications, past test results or treatments. The emergency department may not have access to your doctor's medical records. The information that you take can be extremely important.

The Wise Approach to Surgery

A wise medical consumer approaches any surgery with caution. You will feel better and do better if you know what to expect in advance. Get answers to all ten questions on this page before agreeing to any surgery or major diagnostic procedure.

Second Opinions
If you have doubts about the need for surgery, ask a second doctor to

---

10 Questions to Ask Before Scheduling Surgery

About Your Surgeon:
1. Are you a member of the American College of Surgeons?
2. How many similar surgeries have you performed?

About the Surgery:
3. Is this the usual treatment for my diagnosis? Are there non-surgical treatments?
4. Can a general anesthetic be avoided?
5. What can go wrong? What is the risk of death?
6. How often is the surgery completely successful? What health outcomes should I expect?
7. Does my regular doctor agree that the surgery is needed now?
8. How much will it cost?

About Your Choices:
9. What will happen if I delay or decline the surgery?
10. How can I best prepare for the surgery and the recovery period?

Once you understand the costs, risks, and benefits, surgery becomes your decision.

Surgery - continued

suggest other alternatives. Get an independent opinion. Ask your primary physician, not your surgeon, to recommend another specialist. Also consider getting a second opinion from a different type of physician. If the first doctor is a surgeon, ask a non-surgical specialist who treats similar problems.

Tell the first surgeon that you plan to get a second opinion. Request that your lab results and x-rays be sent to the second physician. Don't pay for the same tests twice.

Save Hospitals for When You Need Them

Save hospitalization for times when you can't get the needed services any other way. If you do need hospitalization, you will be better off to get in and out as quickly as possible. It will cost less and reduce your risk of hospital-induced infections.

Don't check in just for tests. Hospitalization is no longer needed for most medical tests. Ask if the tests can be done on an outpatient basis. If you agree to control your diet and activities, the doctor will usually support your request.

Additional days in the hospital can sometimes be avoided by bringing in extra help at home. Ask about home health nursing services to help while you recover. With such help available, many people can shorten hospital stays.

Hospitals are not the only choice for people with a terminal illness. Many people choose to spend their remaining time at home with people they know and love. Special arrangements for the needed care can be made through hospice care programs in most communities. Try "Hospice" in the Yellow Pages or ask your doctor.

Hospital Consumer Skills

When you need to be in the hospital, good consumer skills can help improve the quality of care you receive. However, don't overdo consumerism. If you are very sick, ask your spouse or a friend to help watch out for your best interests.

- Ask "why?" Don't agree to anything unless you have a good reason. Hospitals have a lot of standard procedures. Agree only to those procedures that make sense for you.

- Provide an extra level of quality control. Check medications, tests, injections, and other treatments to see if they are correct. Your diligence can improve the quality of care that you receive.

- Get personal. Be friendly with the nurses and aides. Friendship both speeds recovery and increases the attention paid to your needs.

- Know your rights. Most hospitals have accepted the "Patient's Bill of Rights" developed by the American Hospital Association. Ask your hospital for a copy.

You Have the Right:

- To be spoken to in words that you understand.

- To be told what's wrong with you.

- To read your medical record.

- To know the benefits and risks of any treatment and its alternatives.

- To know what a treatment or test will cost.

- To make all treatment decisions.

- To refuse any medical procedure.

Eight Ways to Cut Health Care Costs

1. Take good care of yourself.
Eight out of ten health problems are cared for at home, without the help of health professionals. By doing a good job of self-care, you help to reduce costs.

2. Get good professional care.
High quality care costs less than poor quality care. When you improve the quality of your shared treatment plan as described on page 5, you will reduce the cost of care.

3. Reduce your medical test and drug costs.
Ask your doctor about every prescribed medication and medical test. Also ask what will happen if you choose not to take a drug or have a test. Every test and drug has some danger of adverse reactions. Your physician may be able to suggest something less risky.

4. Avoid hospitalization if other options are appropriate.
Over half of all health care costs are for hospitalizations. A stay in a modern hospital costs far more than a vacation at most luxury resorts. (And hospitals are a lot less fun.)

5. Save emergency services for emergencies.
Emergency room services can cost two to three times what the same service costs in a doctor's office.

6. Check your bills.
Hospital bills often contain errors. If you check your bill carefully and notify the hospital and your health plan office of any mistakes, you will help reduce the cost of your health care.

7. Use your health plan resources.
Many health plans now have highly specialized nurses or other professionals available to help you understand and explore alternative treatment plans for major health problems. These people can help you

Cutting Costs - continued

find out the cost, risk, and benefit of most medical tests, surgeries, or other treatments that you may be considering.

8. Avoid defensive medicine.
Defensive medicine refers to tests and services performed primarily to protect physicians from possible malpractice suits. Because every test and procedure has added costs and risks, you may prefer a more conservative approach.

Buying Health Insurance

It is wise to be covered by a good health insurance or health maintenance organization (HMO) plan. Even if you are eligible for Medicare, subscribe to a supplemental policy or plan. One supplemental policy should be all you need. Duplicate insurance policies, especially policies for specific problems like cancer, are usually not in your best interest.

Like Medicare, most standard health plan and health insurance policies do not cover long term care. Whether delivered at home or in a nursing home, long term care services are very expensive. Many insurance companies now offer long term care insurance policies to help protect you against that risk. However, because the long term care insurance field is still new, consumers should be extremely careful to avoid buying something that will not be worth the price.

For good information on long term care insurance, or any kind of health insurance, call the Department of Insurance in your state. They can either help you directly or refer you to someone in your area who can answer questions.

Health Fraud and Quackery

Millions of people are taken in each year by medical fraud and worthless health products. Over 27 billion dollars per year are spent on useless treatments.

A common health fraud is bogus "cures" for chronic problems such as arthritis, cancer, impotence, and baldness. These cures often sound like the only possible answer to your problem. Unfortunately, one out of ten people who try quack remedies is harmed by side effects.

Stay away from products that

- Are advertised by testimonials

- Claim to have a secret ingredient

- Are not evaluated in prominent medical journals

- Claim benefits that seem too good to be true

- Are available only by mail

Principle 4: Trust Your Common Sense

Medicine is not as magical as we once thought. If someone takes the time to explain a problem or a treatment to us, we can usually make a pretty good decision about what is best for us.

The best medical tests, diagnosticians, and medical specialists are not enough. Good medical care also requires your own common sense. If you trust your common sense, you are on your way to becoming a wise medical consumer.

*If I had known I was going to live this long, I would
have taken better care of myself.*
Eubie Blake

2

Prevention and Early Detection

If you practice good prevention, you may never need most of the home treatment guidelines in this book.

Over 50 percent of all health problems are preventable. In most cases, prevention is left entirely up to you. What you eat, how much exercise you get, and how well you follow safety rules will often be enough to avoid a medical problem.

Practicing good prevention does not mean giving up all pleasures. On the contrary, taking pleasure in your life is an important aspect of prevention. A happy person who enjoys a good self-image is generally a healthy person as well.

A Long Healthy Life: Good and Bad News

There is both good news and bad news for older people who want to stay healthy.

First, the bad news: If you start exercising, eating right, relaxing more,

and smoking less, you may extend your life by only a few years or months.

Now, the good news: If you practice good health habits, you will be more active, have fewer illnesses, and enjoy life more during the last five to twenty years of your life.

As much as we wish they would, good health habits do not guarantee a long life. However, they do greatly increase your chances for a good quality of life.

The second piece of good news is that it is never too late to begin. Studies show that no matter how old you are, exercise, good nutrition, and positive expectations can make a big difference in your overall quality of life. You will spend fewer days in bed, nursing homes, and hospitals. You will also have more energy to enjoy doing the things you like most.

A Long Healthy Life - continued

If you stop smoking today, your risk of heart disease is halved within one year. After ten years, your risk of lung cancer drops to half that of a continuing smoker. And, in two days, your kisses will taste much, much better.

If you start eating less fat, you will begin to see reductions in body fat and cholesterol in only a few weeks. Very low-fat diets can actually reverse the process of atherosclerosis.

Changes in levels of physical activity help, too. Beginning even a moderate exercise program can help you feel more energetic after only a few days.

So, don't worry that good health habits won't keep you alive forever. Instead, look forward to having all your future years be good years.

Six Keys to Healthy Aging

There is no magic to vitality and health in old age. Just develop good health habits and stick with them. You will find scores of helpful tips throughout this book. Let these six keys be your general guide.

1. **Take care of your body.**
- Keep physically fit.
   o Do something active every day.
   o Find exercise that you enjoy.
   o Maintain your flexibility, strength, and stamina.

- Eat well.
   o Consume a variety of wholesome foods.
   o Eat less fat and more beans, grains, fruits, and vegetables.
   o Drink lots of water. (Eight 8-ounce glasses of water a day.)

- Recharge your batteries.
   o Get seven to eight hours of sleep per day.
   o Try out a variety of deep breathing and relaxation techniques.

- Don't poison your body.
   o Keep smoke out of your lungs and tobacco out of your mouth.
   o Drink alcohol only in moderation.
   o Avoid unneeded medications.

- Manage illness wisely.
   o Use this book and other resources.
   o Find a good doctor.
   o Maintain control of health care decisions.

2. **Stay mentally active.**
If you want to keep your marbles, use them. The brain benefits from exposure to stimulating environments and activities.

- Learn something new every day.

- Read, write, talk, and think about what interests you.

- Take classes and seminars in new subjects.

3. Nurture the ties that bind.
Studies show that people who have many social ties, such as being married, having contact with friends and relatives, and belonging to a church or social group, have better health than people with few social connections.

- Create a support network of family and friends who will help see you through a crisis.

- Find a friend you can confide in. Be a confidant for someone else.

- Combine physical and social health by joining a walking group or exercise class.

4. Know where your help is.
The best way to stay independent is to know when to ask for help.

- Become familiar with your community's support services for seniors, such as transportation, financial counseling, and meals-on-wheels. The local senior center or Area Agency on Aging is a good place to go for information on available services.

5. Accentuate the positive.
The pictures we have in our minds and the verbal messages or self-talk we give ourselves affect both our minds and bodies.

- Expect good things to happen.

- Add humor, laughter, and fun into every day.

- Count your blessings and express thanks.

6. Celebrate your wisdom.
Victor Hugo said, "One sees a flame in the eyes of the young, but in the eyes of the old, one sees light."
More than anything else, the world needs wisdom.

- Recognize your purpose for living.

- Think about your values and beliefs.

- Help others to gain wisdom, too.

Immunizations

Immunizations provide protection against many serious diseases. Chances are, you have been immunized against the major childhood diseases, or have gained immunity because you had them as a child.

However, there are several immunizations that need to be updated throughout your life. If your doctor does not suggest them to you, make a note to mention them at your next visit.

Older adults need:

- A tetanus booster every ten years.

Immunizations - continued

- An annual influenza shot. (For people over age 65, and those with chronic respiratory problems. See this page.)

- A one-time pneumococcal vaccine. (For anyone age 65 or older, and others at high risk. See this page.)

Tetanus Immunization

Tetanus (lockjaw) is a bacterial infection that is fatal in about 50 percent of cases. The bacteria enter the body through wounds, and thrive only in the absence of oxygen. Puncture wounds, such as from a rusty nail, are especially good environments for the tetanus bacteria, but any cut or scrape can become infected. The only sure protection against tetanus is immunization.

Active immunity is acquired by a basic series of three shots followed by a booster one year later. Routine boosters are then recommended every 10 years throughout your life to maintain immunity. If you have a contaminated wound, you should get another shot if you haven't had one in the past five years.

If you have never been immunized against tetanus, it is a good idea to start the series of three active shots now, then have a booster every 10 years.

Influenza Immunization

Influenza (flu) is a very contagious viral illness that causes fever, aches and pains, sore throat, runny nose, and chills (see page 71).

Older people are more likely to develop complications of influenza, such as pneumonia and dehydration. To protect yourself, get a flu shot each autumn if any of the following applies to you.

- You are over age 65.

- You have diabetes, any immune system disorder, or chronic respiratory problems, such as asthma, bronchitis, or emphysema.

- You are in contact with another person who is ill or has recently been released from the hospital-- this includes children and grandchildren.

Side effects of the flu shot are usually mild, such as a low-grade fever and minor aches. They do not last long.

Do not get a flu shot if you are allergic to eggs. The virus in the vaccine is grown in eggs, and you may develop an allergic reaction. Other medications are available for short-term protection during severe flu outbreaks. Talk with your doctor.

Pneumococcal Immunization

Most people think of pneumococci as the bacteria that cause pneumonia, but they can also cause an infection of the blood (bacteremia) or of the covering of the brain (meningitis). Older people develop pneumococcal infections much more frequently than the general population.

One shot will usually give lifelong protection from pneumococcal infection. Get a pneumococcal vaccine if:

- You are healthy, over 65, and have never received the shot.

- You are under 65, but have heart, kidney, liver, or lung disease, diabetes, Hodgkin's disease, or any immune system disorder. These conditions increase your risk of developing pneumonia. Consult with your doctor.

Side effects of the shot often include mild swelling and pain at the injection site. You can get the pneumococcal vaccine at the same time as one of your yearly flu shots with no adverse effects.

Keep Track of Your Tests and Shots

Plan to keep home medical record files for each member of the family. Keep an immunization and routine test record in front. A list of drugs you are taking is also important. Organize other information by problem. If the problem returns, your record of what happened the last time will be very helpful. See page 342.

Injury Prevention

Accidents do happen, but they don't have to happen to you. Ninety-five percent of all injuries to older adults involve automobile accidents, fires, and falls. Follow these safety precautions to accident-proof your home and yourself.

Automobile Safety Checklist

☐ Always wear a seat belt.

☐ Never drink and drive.

☐ Practice the flexibility exercises on pages 266-275 so you can get the widest range of vision possible.

☐ Check and correct your vision regularly.

☐ Wear good quality sunglasses to reduce glare.

☐ If your night vision is limited, avoid night driving.

☐ If your hearing is limited, keep a window open and the radio down.

☐ Wear light-colored clothing or something reflective when walking at night.

Fire Safety Checklist

☐ Replace frayed or damaged electrical cords.

☐ Remove cords from under rugs and furniture.

☐ Remove nails and staples from all electrical cords.

Fire Safety Checklist - cont'd

- ☐ Check wattage rating of electrical cords and appliances.

- ☐ Install smoke alarms outside bedrooms; at least one per floor.

- ☐ Keep multi-purpose fire extinguishers in the kitchen and near fireplaces or woodstoves.

- ☐ Remove electrical wires that are near tubs, showers, and sinks.

- ☐ Install special safety outlets in your bathroom. Ask for a ground fault circuit interrupter.

- ☐ Don't smoke in bed.

- ☐ Don't tuck electric blankets in or cover them with other blankets.

- ☐ Don't store flammable liquids indoors.

- ☐ Avoid small electric, kerosene, and propane heaters. If you must use them, keep them away from curtains, rugs, and furniture.

- ☐ Follow building codes for installing wood stoves.

- ☐ Clean wood stove or fireplace chimneys at least annually.

- ☐ Keep towels away from the kitchen stovetop.

- ☐ Roll up loose, long sleeves when cooking.

- ☐ Select stovetop controls that clearly show when the heat is on.

- ☐ To avoid burns, set hot water heaters at 120° or lower.

Fall Prevention Checklist

- ☐ Have a lamp or light switch that you can easily reach without getting out of bed.

- ☐ Keep a flashlight handy.

- ☐ Use nightlights in bedroom, bathroom, and in hallways.

- ☐ Have light switches at both ends of stairs and halls.

- ☐ Ensure good lighting in the kitchen and where power tools are used.

- ☐ Use bathmats with suction cups.

- ☐ Sit on a bench or stool in the shower.

- ☐ Add grab bars in shower, tub, and toilet areas.

- ☐ Consider your need for an elevated toilet seat.

- ☐ Install handrails on both sides of stairs.

- ☐ Remove or replace rugs or runners that tend to slip.

- ☐ Wax floors with slip-proof finish.

- ☐ Wear non-slip shoes or slippers.

- ☐ Keep ice cleared from entrances and walks.

- ☐ Remove all clutter from floors and stairways.

- ☐ Keep telephone and electrical cords out of pathways.

- ☐ Tack rugs and glue vinyl flooring so they lie flat.

- ☐ Select carpets with low, tight pile.

☐ Make certain carpet is firmly attached to the stairs.

☐ Purchase a stepstool with high and sturdy handrails. Repair or discard wobbly step-stools.

☐ Paint the edges of outdoor steps and any steps that are especially narrow or are higher or lower than the rest.

☐ Don't wear long skirts or floor-length gowns.

☐ Review medications with your doctor or pharmacist. Some drugs can make you drowsy, dizzy, and unsteady.

☐ Watch alcohol intake. More than two drinks per day can cause unsteadiness.

☐ Have your hearing and eyesight tested. Inner ear problems can affect depth perception and balance. Impaired vision makes it difficult to see potential hazards.

☐ Exercise regularly to improve muscle flexibility and strength.

☐ Learn how to get out of a chair safely (see Sofa Safety on this page and lift objects correctly (See page 35).

For more safety information, see Resource V3 on page 352. For additional auto and driving safety tips, see Resources V1-2 on page 352.

Early Detection

If you can't prevent a health problem, the next best thing is to treat it early. This section provides guidelines for what you and your doctor can do to discover illness while it is easier to treat or cure.

Annual health checkups begin to make sense for women by age 50 and for men by age 65. The chart on the next page suggests which immunizations and tests should be included and how often each should be done. The scientific merit of many of the tests is still under study. Work with your doctor to develop a screening schedule that fits your individual needs and concerns.

Sofa Safety

Many hip fractures happen when older adults with bone or joint problems get up from a sofa or low chair. To reduce your risk of falls and hip fractures, avoid sitting in sofas and chairs that put your hips lower than your knees. Get up from a sofa or chair in the following way:

1. If you are getting up from a sofa, sit next to the arm rest. If the chair has arms, use them for support.

2. Before standing up, put your feet parallel with the toes pointing straight out.

3. Stand slowly, using the arm rest to help you. If the chair doesn't have arm rests, use the edge of the chair.

4. Hold on to the chair or sofa until you have your balance.

Preventive Services Schedule

(Recommended Time Intervals Between Preventive Services[1])

Preventive Service	Age 50-64	Age 65+	Comments
Exams			
Blood pressure p. 86	2-3 years	1 year	Annually, if diastolic pressure is over 85
Blood in stool test p. 98	5 years*	5 years*	More often if relatives have had bowel cancer
Cholesterol p. 288	5 years	5 years	Annually, if last test was over 239 or if high risk for heart disease
Sigmoidoscopy p. 98	10 years*	10 years	More often if relatives have had bowel cancer
Urinalysis p. 347	10 years*	5 years	
Thyroid function p. 127	At age 64	5 years	Annually for all women or men with family history or past upper body radiation
Vision test p. 149	5 years*	5 years	2-3 years with glasses
Glaucoma test p. 154	5 years*	5 years	Every year after age 50 if high risk
Hearing test p. 164	10 years*	5 years	More frequently if hearing problems exist
Dental exam p. 173	6 months	6 months	Plus inspections at home

[1] Adapted from: *Guide to Clinical Preventive Services*, US/DHHS, 1989. The scientific merit of many of the tests is still under study. Work with your doctor to develop a screening schedule that fits your individual needs and concerns.

*Because of insufficient evidence, many experts are uncertain about the effectiveness of regular tests for this age group.

Preventive Services Schedule

(Recommended Time Intervals Between Preventive Services[1])

Preventive Service	Age 50-64	Age 65+	Comments
Immunizations			
Tetanus p. 22	10 years	10 years	Booster shot needed
Influenza p. 22	If high risk	1 year	
Pneumococcal p. 22	If high risk	At age 65	
Women Only			
Breast self-exam p. 205	Monthly*	Monthly*	
Breast exam p. 207	1 year	1 year	
Mammogram p. 207	1-2 years	1-2 years	Uncertain benefits after age 75
Pap smear p. 208	2 years	*	Uncertain benefits after age 65 if previous Pap smears were normal
Men Only			
Prostate exam p. 225	5 years*	5 years*	

[1]Adapted from: *Guide to Clinical Preventive Services*, US/DHHS, 1989. The scientific merit of many of the tests is still under study. Work with your doctor to develop a screening schedule that fits your individual needs and concerns.

*Because of insufficient evidence, many experts are uncertain about the effectiveness of regular tests for this age group.

*I don't deserve this award, but then I have arthritis
and I don't deserve that either.*
Jack Benny

3

Bone, Muscle, and Joint Problems

Bones, muscles, and joints hold you together and allow you to move. As your muscles and bones age, they begin to show signs of wear from a lifetime of use.

- Muscle and bone strength declines.

- Joint flexibility and range of motion declines.

- More pains appear as wear and tear on joints accumulates.

- Muscle quickness diminishes.

Fortunately, you can buck these trends. With regular exercise, good nutrition, and smart home treatment when problems arise, you can expect your body's frame to hold up as long as you do.

Arthritis

Arthritis refers to a variety of joint problems. Simply put, arthritis means inflammation of a joint.

Although arthritis can occur at any age, it affects older people most often.

We know little about what causes most of the 100 different types of arthritis. Certainly, the overuse or abuse of joints can cause arthritis pain in the hands, knees, hips, neck, or back. Heredity also plays a part; arthritis tends to run in families. Certain foods, hormone changes, and immune system problems can also trigger arthritis. Still, how these factors work together to cause problems is largely a mystery.

The table on page 30 describes the four most common kinds of arthritis. Osteoarthritis is by far the most common type for people over 50.

Prevention

There are three keys to preventing further problems associated with arthritis:

- Protect your joints from injury.

Arthritis - continued

- Keep fit.

- Control your weight.

Wear and tear is a frequent factor in arthritis. Overusing a joint can wear it down. Even one day of joint abuse can trigger long-lasting pain. Avoid repeated jarring activities. Stop an activity if you start to feel pain. Don't use aspirin to mask pain while you continue to overuse a fatigued joint.

While wear and tear is bad, regular exercise can be terrific! Stretching maintains your range of pain-free motion. Exercise is needed to nourish the joint cartilage and remove waste products. It also strengthens the muscles around the joint. Strong muscles support the joint and reduce injuries caused by fatigue.

Controlling your weight will also reduce your chances of arthritis pain. Even 10 to 20 extra pounds can add a lot to the load your joints must carry.

Home Treatment

- Follow the Basic Treatment Plan for Arthritis on page 32.

Types of Arthritis			
Type	**Cause**	**Symptoms**	**Comments**
Osteoarthritis	Breakdown of cartilage in joint	Pain, stiffness and swelling of joint	Most common type for both women and men between the ages of 45-90
Rheumatoid Arthritis	Inflammation of the membrane lining the joint	Pain, stiffness, and swelling of joint; fever	Occurs most often in middle age; more common in women
Gout	Build-up of uric acid crystals in the joint fluid	Burning pain, stiffness, and swelling, commonly of the big toe, ankle, knee, wrist, and elbow	Condition may be aggravated by foods high in purines, such as organ meats, or by alcoholic beverages
Ankylosing Spondylitis	Inflammation of ligament at a joint of the spine	Pain and stiffness of the spine	Most common in young men but results of the illness (stiff back) can last a lifetime

- Take advantage of self-help devices that can make everyday chores much easier. See Resource H1 on page 350.

- Learn more about controlling arthritis. See Resource G1 on page 349.

- Avoid arthritis fraud. Mail-order "miracle" cures, secret formulas, and foreign clinics provide no lasting benefit.

- If you regularly suffer from arthritis pain, contact the Arthritis Foundation to learn about their Arthritis Self-Management course.

When to Call a Health Professional

- If you have arthritis pain and fever.

- If the pain is so great that you cannot use the joint.

- If the problem continues for over six weeks and the home treatment is not working. Blood tests can help determine what type of arthritis you have.

- If there is sudden, unexplained swelling, redness, or pain in any joint.

- If arthritis regularly limits your activities, consider seeing a specialist in joint diseases (rheumatologist).

- If you experience side effects of large doses of aspirin or other arthritis medication (nausea, persistent heartburn, or dark tarry stools). See page 336.

- If you experience sudden back pain, see Osteoporosis, page 50.

Joint Replacement Surgery

Sometimes, arthritis will completely destroy a joint. When this happens, the joint can often be surgically replaced. However, joint replacement surgery involves major risks.

Arthritis Success

With arthritis, it helps to look on the bright side. Grandma Moses took up painting at the age of 76 because her arthritis made it too painful to continue with her needlework. She first showed her paintings when she was 80 and continued to paint until she was over 100 years old.

People who decide to take control over their arthritis are usually successful. The more you learn about arthritis, the less it will limit your daily life. Arthritis self-management courses are as effective as most medications available for osteoarthritis.

For help contact your local chapter of the Arthritis Foundation or call (800) 283-7800 for more information.

Basic Treatment Plan for Arthritis

Rest	• Get 8 to 10 hours of sleep per night plus a nap. • See page 302 for a progressive muscle relaxation technique.
Flexibility	• Do the range-of-motion exercises on pages 266 to 275 at least once per day.
Exercise	• Walk at least 30 minutes a day. Work up to that gradually or do it in two or three outings. Wear well-cushioned walking shoes. (Avoid high heels and shoes with pointed toes.) • Water exercises and swimming are easy on the joints. • Stop or change activities if joint pain increases.
Weight Control	• Get closer to your ideal weight. See page 295.
Heat/Cold	• During painful flare-ups, apply moist heat two or three times a day for 20 to 30 minutes. Hot showers, hot soaks, hot packs, or heat lamps can help. Massage sore spots after heat treatments. A warm bath in the morning can help reduce joint stiffness. • Putting cold packs on painful joints can help (10 to 20 minutes at a time). • Try alternating hot and cold treatments.
Water	• Drink two quarts of water per day and eat a well-balanced diet. See page 282.
Medication	• Aspirin can help reduce swelling and ease pain. A coated aspirin at night may reduce joint stiffness in the morning. Be aware of aspirin side effects. See page 336. Stomach bleeding from aspirin overuse is particularly dangerous. Discuss your use of aspirin or other pain relievers with your doctor. • Either aspirin or ibuprofen (Advil) can be helpful, but do not use both in the same day. • Medications can be particularly helpful with rheumatoid arthritis and gout. Ask your doctor.
Observation	• Record any changes that occur in your joints. • Watch to see if sacs of fluid develop behind the knee or under other inflamed joints.

Before agreeing to joint replacement surgery, consider these points:

- Joint replacement surgery is seldom urgent. Get several opinions; a few weeks or months will make little difference. However, the results are often better if the joint is replaced before too much muscle and tendon function have been lost.

- The chance of surgical success is better if you are in good shape. A regular exercise program is critical both before and after the surgery.

- Surgery is most helpful if one joint is causing most of your problems.

- If you have heart or respiratory problems, your risks from surgery are much higher. Tell your surgeon about such problems.

Arthritis Caregiver Tips

- Arthritis pain can cause depression, and depression can increase pain. Review the home treatment for depression on page 240.

- Range-of-motion exercises are very important. Encourage gentle stretching and exercise several times per day.

- Encourage the person with arthritis to do as much for herself as possible. Assistive devices can be helpful. See Resource H1 on page 350.

- Replacement joints do not last forever. A second replacement joint may be needed in 15 to 20 years.

- The surgical risks can be great, the recovery period long, and the pain relief incomplete. Learn the costs, risks, and expected benefits before you agree to joint replacement surgery. See page 13 for "10 Questions to Ask Before Scheduling Surgery."

Back Pain

Your back is made up of the bones of the spine (vertebrae), the discs between the vertebrae, and the muscles and ligaments that hold it all together. Most back trouble involves the discs, muscles or ligaments.

- You can strain your back by overstretching the muscles.

- You can sprain your back by overstretching the ligaments and tendons.

- You can damage your discs so that they rupture or press against a nerve.

Any of these injuries will result in a two or three day period of swelling and acute pain followed by slow healing and a gradual reduction in pain. The goals of self-care are to relieve pain, promote healing, and avoid reinjury.

Back Pain - continued

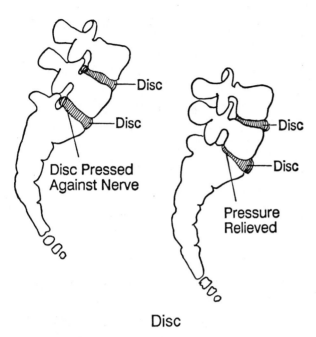

Disc

Ninety percent of back problems can be prevented or remedied with good posture, exercises, and a mix of basic home treatments. Ninety-eight percent of back problems can be successfully treated without surgery.

In addition to the injuries discussed above, back pain can also be caused by arthritis or osteoporosis. Arthritis pain may be a steady ache, unlike the sharp, acute pain of strains, sprains, or disc injury. If you think your back pain may be caused by arthritis, combine the self-care guidelines for back pain with those for arthritis on page 30.

Back pain caused by osteoporosis often comes on suddenly. It is usually caused by a compression fracture of a vertebrae in the middle to lower part of the back. Often there will be no clear reason for the pain. See page 50 for more on osteoporosis.

Quick Reference Guide to Back Pain

- If you have just injured your back by lifting, twisting, bending, or stooping, see the First Aid Guidelines on page 42.

- If you have sudden pain in the middle to lower part of your back, see the section on Osteoporosis on page 50.

- If your pain is due to arthritis, see the Basic Treatment Plan for Arthritis on page 32.

- If you have chronic or recurring back pain, see Home Treatment on page 40.

Prevention

Back Posture
The key to good back posture is keeping the right amount of curve in your lower back. Too much curve ("sway back") or too little curve ("flat back") can result in problems.

Lifting
Follow these tips to avoid compressing the discs of the lower back:

- Bend your knees. Lift with your legs.

- Keep your upper back straight. A slight curve in the lower back is good. One key to preventing back pain is to always maintain a slight arch in your lower back.

- Keep the load as close to your body as possible.

- Never lift from a bent-forward position.

- Avoid turning or twisting your body while holding a heavy object.

- Never lift a heavy object over your head.

Standing

When you stand with good posture, your ear, shoulder, hip, knee, and ankle should all be in a line.

Sitting

When you sit, keep your shoulders back and your lower back supported. Slouching can stress your lower back. Use a small pillow for extra low back support if needed.

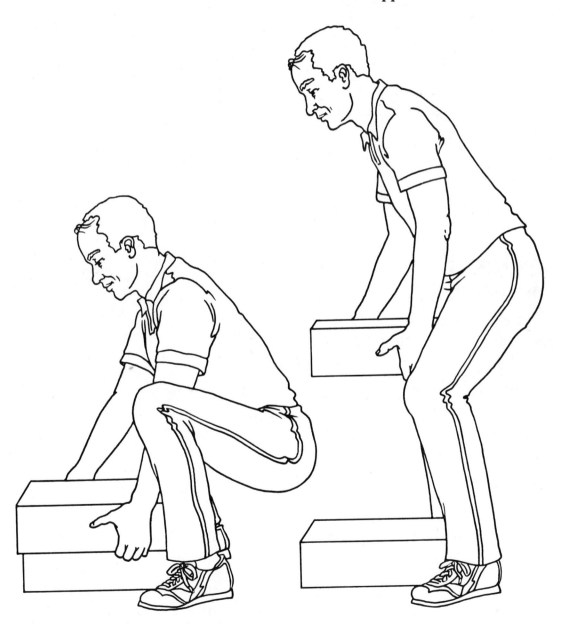

Proper Lifting Posture

Back Pain - continued

Sleeping

A firm bed is best. A sheet of plywood under the mattress may help. Sleep with a slight arch in your lower back.

Exercises To Prevent Back Pain

There are two basic types of exercises that can help your back: extension and flexion. The best type for your back depends on your back pain symptoms. People with healthy backs would do well to practice both types in equal balance.

Extension exercises are designed to strengthen your lower back muscles and to stretch the muscles and ligaments on the stomach side of your back. Extension exercises are particularly helpful if your pain is related to a disc problem.

Flexion exercises are designed to strengthen the stomach muscles and stretch the lower back muscles. They are particularly helpful if your back pain comes from muscle strain, arthritis, or inflammation of the facets where the vertebrae meet.

The Back Pain Exercise Guide on page 39 will help you determine which exercises are best for you. When you are not having back problems, try doing all five exercises every day.

Caution: Let your pain be your guide. A good motto for all the exercises in this chapter is "Strain, not Pain." Some mild strain and discomfort are okay. Stop if you feel sharp pain, or if the discomfort does not improve after the first few minutes of the exercise.

These exercises are not recommended for use during a back pain attack or spasm. Instead, see "First Aid for Back Pain" on page 42.

Basic Extension Exercises

Press-ups

Press-ups can become your basic tool for pain prevention if you have disc-related back pain. Begin and end every set of exercises with a few press-ups (see following page).

- Lie face down with hands at shoulders, palms flat.

- Prop yourself up on your elbows, keeping lower half relaxed.

- Keep hips down and feel a stretch in the lower back.

- Lower to floor and repeat 3 to 10 times, slowly.

Backward Bend

If you need extension exercises, the backward bend can be helpful. Practice it at least once a day and anytime you find yourself working in a bent-forward position.

- Stand upright with your feet slightly apart. (Back up to a counter top for greater support and stability.)

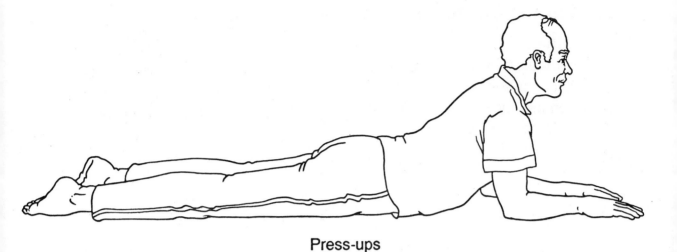

Press-ups

- Keep your knees straight and bend only at the waist.

- Place your hands in the small of your back and gently bend backward.

- Hold the backward stretch for one to two seconds.

- Repeat five times, bending a little farther each time.

Shoulder Lifts

Shoulder lifts will strengthen the back muscles that support the spine (see following page).

- Lie face down with your arms beside your body.

- Lift your head and shoulders straight up from the floor as high as your pain allows.

- Start with five repetitions. Add one per day until you can comfortably do 20.

- Stop if you experience increasing pain.

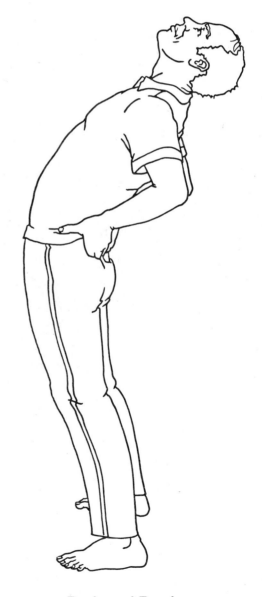

Backward Bend

Basic Flexion Exercises

Knee to Chest

The knee-to-chest exercise stretches the low back muscles and relieves pressure on the bone facets where the vertebrae come together.

- Lie on your back with knees bent and feet close to buttocks.

- Bring your knees to your chest, pulling them as close as possible with your hands. Hold for ten seconds.

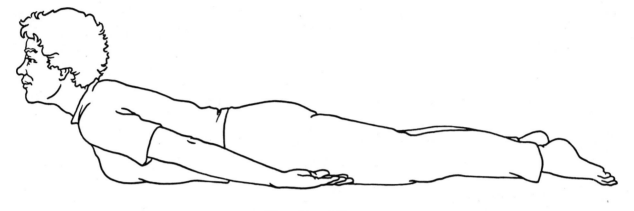

Shoulder Lifts

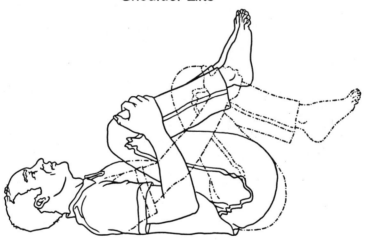

Knee to Chest Exercise

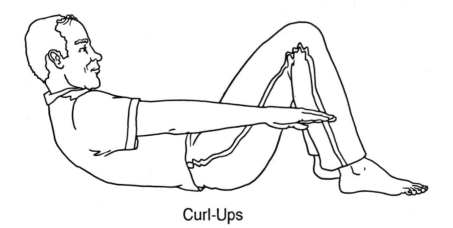

Curl-Ups

- Relax and lower to starting position.

- Repeat five times.

- Stop if you experience increasing pain.

Curl-ups

Curl-ups (illustrated on the previous page) are good exercises for strengthening your abdominal muscles, which work with your back muscles to support your spine.

- Lie on your back with knees bent (60-degree angle) and feet flat on floor.

- Reach for your knees with your hands while tucking your chin and lifting your shoulders up. Keep your lower back pressed to the floor. To avoid neck problems, remember to lift your shoulders and not force your head up and forward.

- Do this exercise slowly.

Back Pain Exercise Guide

Use this guide to help determine whether the flexion or extension exercises on pages 36 to 39 will be most helpful for you.

Symptom of back pain	Flexion	Extension
Sitting or Standing		
Hurts more when sitting		✓
Hurts more when standing	✓	
Morning or Evening		
Hurts more in the morning		✓
Hurts more in the evening	✓	
Stooping or Reaching		
Hurts when bending or stooping		✓
Hurts when reaching or stretching	✓	
Active or Inactive		
Hurts more after being inactive		✓
Hurts more after being active	✓	
Low Back or Abdominal Weakness		
Low back weakness		✓
Abdominal weakness	✓	

Flexion Exercises - continued

- DO NOT HOOK YOUR FEET UNDER ANYTHING.

- Start with five repetitions, increasing one per day until you can comfortably do 20.

- Stop if you experience increasing pain.

General Exercise

Walking, swimming, and biking are all excellent ways to maintain cardiovascular fitness. With good shoes and good techniques that maintain a slight curve in the lower back, aerobic exercise will also contribute to a healthy back.

If any exercise causes increasing or continuing back pain, stop the exercise until you can reevaluate both your back pain and your exercise technique.

Golf, tennis, bowling, aerobic dance, and weight lifting all involve awkward movements of the back. You can participate in these activities without pain if you avoid awkward motions and alter your techniques to stabilize your lower back and maintain a slight curve.

Exercises to avoid:

- Straight leg sit-ups

- Bent leg sit-ups during acute back pain

- Legs up (lifting both legs while lying on your back)

- Heavy weight lifting above the waist

Home Treatment for Back Pain

- As soon as you feel a slip or catch in your back, follow the "First Aid for Back Pain" guidelines on page 42.

- Repeat the exercises every two to three hours for the rest of the day. Avoid any exercise that increases the pain.

- Apply cold packs over the next few days. Twenty minutes every waking hour is good.

- Use aspirin or other pain relievers sensibly. Too much pain relief may allow movement that will worsen the injury.

- Do what you can to relax your muscles. See page 302 for progressive muscle relaxation.

- Avoid any awkward movements and maintain perfect posture. Support your lower back.

- After a week or two of progressive recovery, return to the prevention exercises on page 36.

When to Call a Health Professional

- If you have severe pain in the leg that extends below the knee.

- If you have weakness, numbness, or tingling in the foot and toes.

- If low back pain follows a recent fall or accident.

- If you feel ill or feverish.

- If you have difficulty urinating.

- If you have chronic back pain and the home treatment and prevention guidelines do not help.

- If you develop a new pain in your lower back that does not increase with movement and is not related to stress or muscle tension-- to rule out an aortic aneurysm (weakened, dilated area of an artery).

- If you are now in severe pain, call your doctor. If professional help is needed, ask if a house call is possible. The car trip to the doctor's office can worsen a back injury.

Who to See and What to Expect

Medical Doctors

In addition to diagnosing the cause of back pain and evaluating back injuries, a medical doctor can also:

- Prescribe muscle relaxants, anti-inflammatory drugs, and pain relievers.

- Refer you to a physical therapist.

- Recommend back surgery.

Note: If you do get a strong pain-killer or muscle relaxer, take special care to avoid re-injuring your back.

Physical Therapists

After the initial first-aid actions, a physical therapist with training in orthopedic treatment can help you:

- Identify specific muscle or disc problems.

- Help you improve your posture and customize an exercise program for recovery and long-term protection.

- Provide short-term relief with massage or other therapies.

Other Professionals

Chiropractors, acupuncturists, massage therapists, and others may also offer short-term relief.

Back Surgery

Doctors recommend back surgery much less frequently now than in the past. Rest, posture changes, and exercise can relieve 90 percent of back problems.

If home treatment and conservative medical treatment do not work, take some time to consider your options. Before you agree to back surgery, get good answers to the ten questions on page 13.

Even as a last resort, surgery often fails to improve back problems.

First Aid For Back Pain

When you first feel a catch or slip in your back, there are four things you can do to avoid or reduce expected pain. **Stop any exercise if the pain becomes severe or increases.**

First Aid # 1 : Backward Bend

Stand with hands on hips and stretch backwards. Hold the stretch for two seconds.

First Aid # 2: Squat

Go into a flat-footed squat (20 to 40 seconds). Don't bounce. Don't stand up from the squat; go directly to First Aid #3.

First Aid # 3: Relax

Lie flat on your stomach with your arms beside your body and your head to one side (one to two minutes).

First Aid # 4: Prop Up

Prop yourself up on your elbows with your forearms in front. Partially arch your back (two to five minutes).

First Aid # 5: Ice

As soon as possible, apply ice, not heat, to an injured back. Ice or cold packs will limit swelling, reduce pain, and speed healing.

If you successfully complete all five first aid actions, continue with the home treatment guidelines.

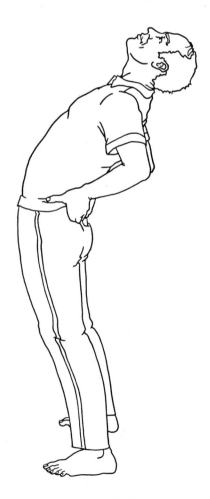

First Aid #1

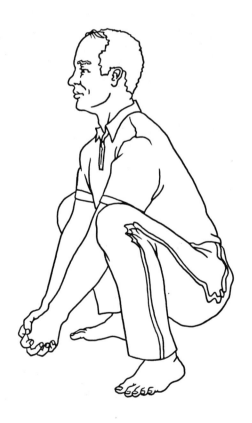

First Aid #2

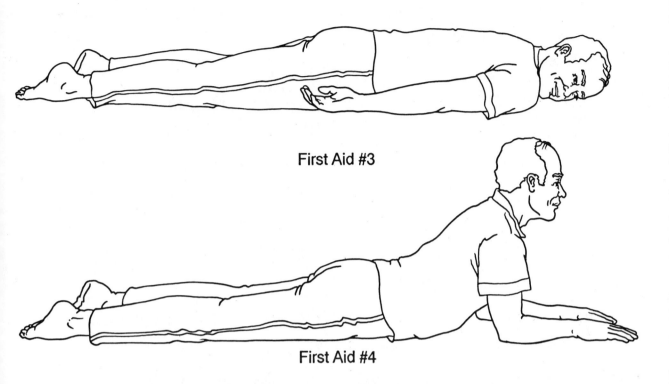

First Aid #3

First Aid #4

Bunions and Hammer Toes

A bunion is a swelling of the foot at the base of the big toe. An acute bunion is a type of bursitis; the bursa covering the big toe joint becomes inflamed and painful.

Hammer toes are toes that bend down permanently at a middle joint. Both conditions are usually caused by wearing shoes that are too short or too narrow.

Prevention

- Wear shoes that do not squeeze or rub on your toes. Shoes that are too short or that have pointed toes may cause bunions and hammer toes.

Home Treatment

Once you have a bunion or hammer toe, there is usually no way to completely get rid of it, short of surgery.

- Avoid shoes that are too tight, too short, or that have high heels. Custom-made shoes are an option if your bunion is very painful, but they are quite expensive.

- Wear sandals or other shoes that do not put pressure on the bunion or hammer toe.

- Cut out the area over the bunion or hammer toe from an old pair of sneakers or shoes to wear around the house.

- Cushion the bunion or hammer toe with felt, moleskin, or padding to prevent rubbing and irritation.

Bunions - continued

- Try aspirin or ibuprofen (Advil) to relieve pain.

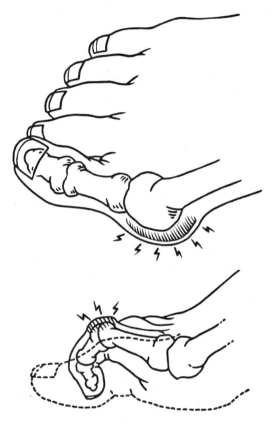

Bunion and Hammer Toe

When to Call a Health Professional

- If walking is extremely difficult or painful. Your doctor may be able to inject the bunion or hammer toe with cortisone to relieve the inflammation. Surgery to align the big toe or straighten the hammer toe may be needed in severe cases.

- If you have diabetes or peripheral vascular disease and a bunion or hammer toe becomes inflamed or irritated. The risk of infection is high for people with these conditions. Good foot care is very important. See page 122.

Bursitis

A bursa is a small sac of fluid that helps the muscles to slide easily over other muscles or bones. Injury or long-term wear and tear of the bursa results in localized pain and inflammation. This condition is known as bursitis.

Bursitis usually develops quickly, over no more than a few days, often as a result of a specific injury. Tennis elbow, frozen shoulder, housemaid's knee, and similar local soreness problems all involve some form of bursitis.

Bursitis in the wrist can cause nerve pressure and pain known as carpal tunnel syndrome. See page 45. A similar problem called Morton's neuroma causes numbness in the front (top) of the foot.

Prevention

The first case of bursitis may be difficult to prevent. Knee pads, good tennis instruction (two-handed backhand stroke), and sensible activities will certainly help. Prevent additional flare-ups by avoiding the activities that cause the problem.

To avoid Morton's neuroma, follow the home treatment guidelines for bursitis and avoid wearing tightly fitting shoes.

Home Treatment

If left alone, bursitis will usually go away or subside in a few days or weeks.

- Rest the inflamed joint. Avoid the original cause of the injury as long as possible even after the pain subsides. Use a sling to support an elbow or shoulder for a day or two.

- Apply ice as soon as you notice the problem. Use ice bags or cold packs for 15 minute periods, twice an hour for six to twelve hours. Heating pads and hot baths will feel good, but ice or cold packs will speed healing.

- Aspirin may help, but don't overdo it. See page 336.

- Gently move the joint through its full range of motion several times a day to prevent stiffness. Gradually increase the exercise to rebuild muscle strength.

When to Call a Health Professional

- If there is fever of 101° or higher, redness, or an inability to use the joint (to rule out a bacterial infection).

- If the problem is severe and you can think of no injury or activity that may have caused it.

- If the pain persists for two weeks or longer. Your physician can help you develop a new home treatment plan. Corticosteroid drugs can be injected for severe cases. Be sure to ask about the risks and alternatives before agreeing to treatment.

Carpal Tunnel Syndrome

Bursitis, arthritis, or injury to the wrist can create a secondary problem called carpal tunnel syndrome. Swelling in the inflamed ligament squeezes the median nerve as it passes through the carpal tunnel in the front of the wrist.

Symptoms include pain in the wrist, shooting pain up to the elbow or down to the fingers, and numbness in all but the little finger.

Home Treatment

- Avoid repetitive hand motions with a bent wrist. Find ways to write, type, paint, play piano, etc. with your wrist in a neutral (straight) position. If symptoms lessen, gradually resume the activity and try to keep the wrist straight.

- Decrease inflammation with aspirin or ibuprofen (Advil).

- A wrist splint may help, especially if worn at night. Get one from your pharmacy or a hospital supply store.

Gout

Gout is a form of arthritis caused when uric acid crystallizes in the joints. The cause of gout is well-known and the treatment is highly effective.

Gout attacks can come on suddenly. The pain often reaches its peak in a matter of hours. The joint becomes tender, swollen, red, and extremely painful. A low fever of 99° to 100° is common.

Gout is far more common in men than in women. Most of the time it attacks the joint of the big toe first. If gout is not treated when it first occurs, elbows, ankles, knees, fingers, and other joints may be involved in later attacks.

Gout attacks can last from several days to weeks. Between attacks, months or years can go by with no symptoms. Attacks gradually increase in frequency, duration, and severity.

Prevention

If you are prone to gout attacks:

- Avoid or cut back on wine, beer, and other alcoholic beverages. Excessive drinking is particularly harmful.

- Avoid gravy, organ meats, sardines, mussels, scallops, and anchovies. Cut back on dried peas, legumes, and other foods rich in purines.

- Avoid excessive use of aspirin.

- Drink lots of water to flush the uric acid out of your system. Two quarts per day (eight 8-ounce glasses) would be great.

- Control your weight. See page 295. Weight control is sometimes the only treatment needed for gout.

Home Treatment

- Avoid aspirin products. They can cause a build-up of uric acid. Reduce gout pain with acetaminophen (Tylenol) or with ibuprofen (Advil), which also reduce inflammation. People with high blood pressure, heart disease, or kidney problems should consult their doctors before using ibuprofen.

- Use anti-gout medications as prescribed by a physician. Many of these drugs have severe side effects. Avoid using more than prescribed. Stop taking the drug and call your doctor if reactions such as nausea, vomiting, diarrhea, or abdominal cramping appear.

- Diuretic medications (water pills) prescribed for high blood pressure can complicate gout. Ask if an alternative would be appropriate.

- Create a tent over your toe or joint to reduce pressure from bed sheets.

- Wear sandals.

- Drink even more water. Aim for three quarts a day.

When to Call a Health Professional

- Call a doctor anytime you suspect gout to be the problem.

- There are two main types of gout medications. One type is used to treat acute gout attacks. It can provide nearly complete gout pain relief within a few hours. The second type of medication prevents gout by lowering the levels of uric acid. Once started, long-term treatment is required.

Joint Infections

Infections from illnesses elsewhere in the body can spread to joints and bones. People using steroid medications or who have a lower resistance to infection for other reasons are at particular risk.

The infection can be viral, bacterial, or fungal. Staph infections, rheumatic fever, and even Lyme disease are examples.

When to Call a Health Professional

Joint and bone infections, sometimes called septic arthritis, can often be cured with medications. Call your doctor promptly if any of these symptoms cause you to suspect an infection:

- Sudden onset of pain in joints without known injury

- Joint pain with fever and chills

- Any joint that is painful, swollen, warm, and inflamed (red) without known injury

- Joint pain associated with symptoms of infection in the lungs or elsewhere

Leg Pain

Leg and muscle cramps are common in older adults. They are often caused by low levels of calcium in the blood. Leg pain can also be due to phlebitis, an inflammation of a vein in the leg. See page 90.

Pain in your shin may be caused by an irritation of the tissues that hold the leg muscle to the bone. This condition is called shin splints, and may occur soon after you start an exercise program.

Prevention

- Get regular exercise during the day and do stretching exercises just before bedtime.

- Include plenty of calcium in your diet or take calcium supplements. See page 292.

- Take a warm bath before bedtime.

- Keep legs warm while sleeping.

Leg Pain - continued

- Try elastic stockings during the day.

- Don't smoke.

Home Treatment

- If there is heaviness and pain deep in the leg, call your doctor before applying home treatment.

- Ask someone to rub or knead a cramping muscle while you stand. Don't rub if you suspect a blood clot.

- Use a heating pad or hot pack to warm the cramping muscle.

- Follow the prevention guidelines.

- Shin splints are best treated with ice, aspirin, and a week or two of rest followed by a gradual return to low-impact exercise (swimming, walking, biking). If healing is slow, consider the home treatment advice for stress fractures on page 53.

When To Call a Health Professional

If you have the following symptoms of phlebitis:

- Heaviness and pain deep in the leg

- Unexplained swelling and redness in one leg

- Shortness of breath or chest pain (Emergency Situation)

- Leg cramps that worsen or persist in spite of prevention and home treatment

Neck Pain

Neck pain and stiffness is usually caused by strained or cramped neck muscles. Neck movement may be limited, usually more to one side than the other. Headaches often come with neck pain.

Neck muscle strain can be due to any of the following:

- Sleeping on a pillow that's too high

- Poor posture

- Extended periods of "the thinker's pose" (resting your forehead on your upright fist or arm)

- Other pressures on the neck muscles

- Any blow directly to the neck or any sudden movement that snaps or jerks the neck

Meningitis, a life-threatening condition, causes a severe stiff neck with headache and fever. If these three symptoms come together, you should see a doctor promptly.

Prevention

- If neck stiffness is worse in the morning, improve your sleeping support. A hard mattress or a special "neck support" pillow may solve the problem. Fold a towel lengthwise into a four-inch pad. Wrap it around your neck and pin it for good support.

- If neck pain is worse at the end of the day, review your posture and body mechanics during daily activities. Avoid supporting your head with your hand.

- Strengthen and protect your neck by doing the following prevention exercises. Stop any exercise that causes sharp pain.

1. Sit or stand erect in a "palace guard" posture (chin in, chest out). Hold for a count of five; then relax. Repeat six times. This stretches the back of the neck.

2. Starting from the palace guard posture, gently drop your head backward. Repeat six times.

3. Gently squeeze your shoulders together six times.

4. Move your head backward, forward, and side-to-side against gentle pressure from your hands. Repeat six times.

5. Do six shoulder lifts as shown on page 38.

Home Treatment

- Place a cold pack over painful muscles for 10 to 15 minutes at a time. You can do this as often as once an hour. This will help decrease any pain, muscle spasm, or swelling that may be the result of an injury.

- If swelling is not a problem, heat may also be helpful.

- Gentle exercises can be very helpful. Do the prevention exercises every two to three hours. Stop doing any exercise that causes sharp pain.

- Aspirin can help relieve pain. Prescription anti-inflammatory medications may also be helpful in reducing swelling in the damaged tissue.

When to Call a Health Professional

If you can't touch your chin to your chest or if stiffness, headache, and fever are present. A spinal tap may be required to rule out meningitis. The more severe the symptoms, the faster you should act.

- If the pain extends or shoots down one arm or you have numbness or tingling in your hands. An x-ray may be needed to rule out a pinched nerve. Muscle relaxants may be prescribed. See page 10 for questions to ask about x-rays.

- If the pain is becoming chronic (two weeks or longer) and the home care does not seem to help. A physician or physical therapist skilled in working with orthopedic problems can help you to develop a treatment plan.

Neck Pain - continued

- If a blow or injury to the neck has caused acute pain.

Osteoporosis

Osteoporosis or "brittle bones" is a condition that affects 25 percent of women over 60 years old. Osteoporosis is less common and less severe in men. It is caused by loss of bone mass and bone strength. It can lead to serious problems with broken arms, legs, hips, and vertebrae. Bone mass declines more quickly in women after menopause when estrogen levels drop.

Other risk factors for osteoporosis include thin body frame, sedentary lifestyle, and a family history of brittle bone fractures. Those who drink or smoke are at greater risk. To assess your personal risk, see "What Are Your Risks of Osteoporosis?" on the next page.

Osteoporosis is a silent disease; there are no symptoms until a bone breaks and the condition is recognized after x-rays. The first indication may be hip or low back pain or painful swelling of a wrist after a minor fall.

X-rays that measure bone density are available. These may be especially useful for women at high risk of osteoporosis in determining who will benefit from estrogen replacement therapy. Estrogen helps bones absorb calcium. Ask your doctor about your need for this test.

Prevention

- Get regular, weight-bearing exercise, such as walking, bicycle riding, or dancing. Bones get stronger with exercise. See page 255.

- Add calcium to your diet. The average American diet contains 500 mg. After menopause, women need about 1500 mg. The extra 1000 mg can come from a large increase in dairy products or from calcium supplements. One quart of skim milk would add about 1100 mg of calcium. Five 500 mg tablets of calcium carbonate (TUMS) will add about 1000 mg of calcium. Take a few tablets with each meal or with milk. Don't take them all at once. Because too much calcium carbonate can cause constipation, limit yourself to no more than eight TUMS per day and drink lots of water.

- Consider small supplements of vitamin D if you do not get enough sunshine for your body to make its own. However, since too much vitamin D (more than 1000 I.U. per day) is harmful, consult a registered dietitian or your doctor first.

- Don't smoke.

- Drink alcohol in moderation.

What Are Your Risks of Osteoporosis?

Risk Factors: Circle points that apply to you.

Age 35-64	2
Age 65-79	5
Age 80 +	8
Caucasian or Asian	2
Small-boned	2
Slender	2
Mother, grandmother, or sister with osteoporosis	2
Post-menopausal	1
Hysterectomy	1
Never been pregnant	1
Have breast-fed	1
Allergic to milk	1
Smoker	1
Over 4 caffeinated colas or coffees per day	1
Over 1 ounce of alcohol per day	1

Risk Factor Score (Add risk factor points.) .... _____

Prevention Factors: Circle points that apply to you.

Exercise (walking or equivalent)

Walk 1/2-1 miles a day	1
Walk 1-2 miles a day	2
Walk 3+ miles a day	3

Diet

1000-1500 mg of calcium per day	1
1500+ mg of calcium per day	2
Receive estrogen replacement therapy	2
30 minutes of sunshine per day or 400 International Units of Vitamin D	1

Prevention Factor Score (Add prevention points.) .... _____

Subtract Prevention Factor Score from Risk Factor Score

Osteoporosis Risk Predictor .... _____

Score Interpretation

Low Risk: Less than 9   High Risk: 16-20

Medium Risk: 9-15   Very High Risk: 21+

Osteoporosis - continued

- Consider estrogen replacement therapy if you are at high risk for osteoporosis or if you have had a brittle bone fracture. See page 211 for the risks and benefits of estrogen replacement therapy.

Home Treatment

- Follow the prevention guidelines above.

- Because prolonged inactivity produces rapid bone loss, remain as active as possible following a brittle bone fracture or any extended period of bed rest.

- For collapsed vertebrae, a back brace can help you remain active during the six to eight week healing period.

- Work with a physical therapist to develop an exercise plan.

- See the Fall Prevention Checklist on page 24.

When to Call a Doctor

- If you experience a fall resulting in hip pain or are unable to get up after a fall.

- If you have sudden, unexplained pain in your back that does not improve after two to three days of home treatment.

- To discuss estrogen replacement therapy. See page 211.

Strains, Sprains, and Fractures

A **strain** is an injury caused by over-stretching a muscle.

A **sprain** is an injury to the muscle and the ligaments, tendons, or soft tissues around a joint. Generally, sprains hurt more and last longer than strains. However, the treatment is usually the same.

A **fracture** is a broken bone. Most fractures also involve strains and sprains to the connecting muscles and ligaments. In stress fractures, the break may be nothing more than a tiny crack.

Stress fractures are often due to a sudden increase in exercise that pounds the bones. While all fractures need to be seen by a physician, minor breaks can usually wait a while. Call your doctor before rushing to an emergency room.

Taking the time for good home treatment will often prevent further damage to an injured limb on the way to see the doctor.

Prevention

Most sprains, strains, and fractures in older adults are the result of falls. To reduce the chance of falls, follow the Fall Prevention Checklist on page 24.

Home Treatment

- Apply ice immediately. Cold will reduce swelling and pain. Apply for 20 minute periods as often as you like for the first 24 hours.

- Splint or wrap an injured joint to prevent movement and additional injury.

- Completely rest the injured area for at least a day. Elevate the injured area if possible. Put no weight on an injured joint for at least a day.

- Take aspirin or ibuprofen (Advil) to help reduce pain. However, don't mask the pain and continue to use the injured joint.

- **For foot or ankle:**

  - Use crutches or a wheelchair for a few days to speed healing.

  - For chronic strain of the muscles at the balls of your feet, avoid long walks or jogging for several weeks. After the foot heals, gradually increase exercise and wear well-cushioned shoes.

  - For a stress fracture to the foot, use crutches until the pain subsides and treat the foot gently for six weeks or more. You will not usually need a cast.

Removing a Ring

To remove a ring from a sprained or swollen finger:

- First, try soapy water. Ice water will also decrease the swelling.

- Stick the end of a slick piece of string or dental floss under the ring toward the hand.

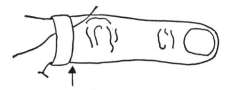

Start Wrapping Here

- Starting at the knuckle side of the ring, wrap the string snugly around the finger toward the end of the finger. Wrap beyond the knuckle. Each wrap should be right next to the one before.

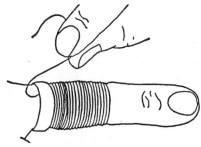

- Grasp the end of the string that is stretched under the ring and start unwrapping it. Push the ring along to take the place of the unwrapped string until the ring passes the knuckle.

Strains, Sprains - continued

- Do exercises that do not put stress on the injured bone. Swimming and bike riding are good.

- **For hands or fingers:**

  - If the injury is to a finger or hand, immediately remove all rings. See page 53. Rings may have to be cut off after swelling occurs.

- **For knees:**

  - For a sprained knee, follow the basic home treatment. Add stretches to avoid chronic knee stiffness. A gradual return to exercise can include swimming, biking, and walking with well-cushioned shoes.

- **For back and neck:**

  - For sprains and strains of the back, see page 33.

  - For sprains and strains of the neck, see page 48.

When to Call a Health Professional

- You may have broken a bone if:

  - A limb is twisted or bent out of shape.

  - A bone is poking through the skin.

  - You cannot move the injured limb.

  - You can feel a bump or irregularity along the bone line. Gently press the injured area. Pain is often centered at the site of a break. Pain from a sprain is usually more spread out.

- If there is a lot of swelling and bruising.

- If hip, low back, or wrist pain develops after a fall. Even minor falls can break bones weakened by osteoporosis.

- If the pain increases after home treatment.

- If a sprain does not improve after four days of home treatment.

Tendinitis

Tendons are the tough, rope-like fibers that connect muscles to bones. Tendinitis is an inflammation of the tendons and their attachments to the bones and muscles. Generally, the home treatment for tendinitis is the same as for bursitis (rest, ice, aspirin, and range-of-motion exercises). See page 45.

If the injury is to the Achilles tendon (the tendon above the heel), add gentle stretching to the tendon after a week of self-care.

If the injury is to the tendons around the shoulder, gradually add weights after a week of the range-of-motion exercises.

Weakness and Fatigue

Weakness is a physical inability or difficulty in moving an arm or leg or other muscle.

Fatigue is a feeling of tiredness, exhaustion, or listlessness.

Unexplained muscle weakness is serious. It is often due to metabolic problems such as diabetes (page 120), thyroid problems (page 126), or kidney problems (page 116). An immediate call to your doctor is appropriate.

Fatigue, on the other hand, can usually be treated well with self-care. Most problems with fatigue are caused by lack of exercise, depression, worry, or boredom. Colds and flu may sometimes cause fatigue and weakness, but the symptoms disappear as the illness runs its course.

Prevention

- Regular exercise is the best defense against fatigue. If you feel too tired to exercise, a short walk is probably the best thing you can do.

- Eat a well-balanced diet. Also consider a basic vitamin supplement as discussed on page 292.

- Improve your sleeping habits. See page 251.

- Deal with any depression over a loss. See page 240.

Home Treatment

- Follow the prevention guidelines above and be patient. It may take a while to feel energetic again.

- Listen to your body. Alternate rest with exercise.

- Limit drugs that might contribute to fatigue. Tranquilizers and cold and allergy medications are particularly suspect.

- Reduce your use of caffeine, nicotine, and alcohol.

- Cut back on television and replace it with new activities, friends, or travel to break the fatigue cycle.

When to Call a Health Professional

- Immediately, if you have severe muscle weakness that you cannot explain.

- If you have experienced sudden, unplanned weight loss.

- If, in spite of home treatment, you are unable to do your usual activities.

- If, after six weeks of home treatment, you do not feel more energetic.

Dealing with Chronic Pain

There is no magic solution to chronic pain, whether it is caused by arthritis, back problems, cancer, or any other illness. No one can offer complete and total relief. However, the following tips may help.

1. **Experiment with heat, cold, and massage.** Find out what works best for you. Touch is important, too. Ask for and give lots of hugs.

2. **Continue to exercise.** Find enjoyable exercise that does not aggravate the pain. Use the stretching exercises on pages 266 to 275 every day.

3. **Try to relax.** Severe pain makes your body tense and tight, and the tension may make the pain worse. See the relaxation techniques on page 300. It takes practice to learn any relaxation skill. Give a method a two-week trial. If it doesn't work for you, try another.

4. **Do something distracting.** Focusing all your attention on the pain makes it seem all-consuming. Refocus your attention away from the pain and onto something else. Sing a song, recite a poem, or concentrate on a visualization. See page 308.

5. **Expose yourself to humor.** A good, hearty belly laugh can provide your body with natural pain relief. Laughter **is** the best medicine.

6. **Practice positive self-talk.** Refuse to entertain negative, self-defeating thoughts or feelings of hopelessness. See page 307.

7. **Join a support group.** By being around others who share your problem, you and your family can learn skills for coping with pain. To find a group near you, contact the American Chronic Pain Association, P.O. Box 850, Rocklin, CA 95677 (916) 632-0922.

8. **Consider going to a pain clinic.** Be wary of those that promise complete relief from pain or that use only one method of treatment. Approved programs are registered with the Commission on Accreditation of Rehabilitative Facilities (CARF), 2500 N. Pantano Road, Tucson, AZ 85715, (602)748-1212.

9. **Appeal to the Spirit.** If you believe in a higher power, ask for support and relief from the pain.

10. **Get educated.** See Resource U 1 on page 352 for a book that deals with chronic pain control.

Keep breathing.
Sophie Tucker

4

Chest, Lung, and Respiratory Problems

This chapter will help you respond to the symptoms of respiratory problems. Most respiratory problems are viral infections like colds and flu that usually get better on their own. Good self-care for these minor ailments helps prevent more serious complications.

If more serious problems do develop, the guidelines in this chapter will help you identify them early. Prompt medical treatment from your doctor and from you will often keep even major problems from getting out of hand.

Allergies/Hay Fever

Allergies come in many forms. Hay fever, with its symptoms of itchy watery eyes, sneezing, runny or stuffy nose, temporary loss of smell, and headache, is the most common allergy. Dark rings under the eyes, called "allergic shiners," may also

develop due to restricted blood flow near the sinuses.

In adults, hay fever is caused by dust or plant pollen, particularly ragweed. Animal dander, feathers, mold and mildew, or the mites that live in household dust can also bring on an allergy attack. Allergies seem to run in families. It is possible to develop hay fever at any age. Suspect an allergy if you have a cold that comes seasonally or that seems to linger on and on.

Prevention

- If you know the cause of an allergic reaction, you can prevent allergy attacks by avoiding the plants, animals, or chemicals that create the problem.

- Keep a diary of all contacts--plants, dust, animals, chemicals--and relate these to the symptoms.

Allergies - continued

- Wear a mask/filter while housecleaning or cutting grass.

- Keep the home as dust-free as possible. Change all heating and air conditioning filters monthly.

- In the bedroom, use synthetic pillows and plastic covers on mattresses and pillows.

- Wash bedding weekly.

- Eliminate perfumes, room deodorizers, cleaning products, and other products which may add to the problem.

- Keep pets out of the bedroom.

Home Treatment

- Antihistamines may relieve symptoms. Use caution when taking these drugs. See page 333.

- Get extra rest during an allergy attack.

When to Call a Health Professional

- If the allergy causes severe breathing difficulty or wheezing.

- If there is facial or ear pain.

- If nasal discharge turns green or yellow.

- To get help in identifying the cause of the allergy.

- If symptoms seem worse over time, you and your doctor can consider shots. Allergy shots may help to reduce sensitivity to the allergen. However, you may later develop allergies to different things, or you may move to an area with different irritants.

Asthma

Asthma is the Greek word for panting. Someone having an asthma attack is literally panting for breath. Asthma is a chronic condition of recurrent, reversible obstruction of the airways. The muscles surrounding the air tubes of the lungs go into spasm, the mucous lining swells, and secretions build up. Breathing becomes quite difficult.

Asthma usually happens in attacks or episodes. During an episode, the person may make a whistling or wheezing sound while breathing. The wheeze can be heard some distance away. The person usually coughs a great deal and may spit up mucus.

Asthma is not often fatal. It is serious, however, and in recent years the number of deaths has risen. A severe attack may be effectively treated by inhaled medications and, at times, injections.

Asthma may appear for the first time in adulthood, often during or following a case of the flu or a bad cold. This type of asthma is not seasonal; the attacks occur throughout the year.

Adults who develop asthma can also become sensitive to chemicals and pollutants. The symptoms are the same: wheezing, coughing, and shortness of breath.

Common asthma triggers include: air pollution; colds or the flu; exercise; analgesics (especially aspirin); food preservatives and dyes; emotional stress; animal hair and dander; pollen; dust; smoke; and vapors from household products.

Prevention

No one knows for sure how to prevent asthma from developing. However, if you do have asthma, you can help prevent asthma attacks by avoiding allergens and by strengthening your lungs.

- Asthma attacks are usually triggered by something around you to which you are allergic or sensitive. Discover and avoid the things that cause your asthma attacks.

  - Avoid smoke of all kinds. Stop smoking. Eat, work, travel, and relax in smoke-free areas.

  - Avoid air pollution. Stay indoors on days when the air pollution is high.

  - Avoid breathing cold air. In cold weather, breathe through your nose and cover your nose and mouth with a scarf or a cold weather mask. Masks are available at most drug stores.

  - Reduce your risks of colds and flu by washing your hands often and getting a flu shot each year.

  - Review and follow the prevention guidelines for allergies on page 57.

- Build up the strength of your lungs and airways.

  - Try pursed-lip breathing exercises (see below).

  - Practice roll breathing exercises as described on page 300.

Pursed-Lip Breathing*

Pursed-lip breathing helps release stale air trapped deep in your lungs. Practice the exercise three times a day and at the first indication that airway problems are limiting your breathing.

1. Relax your body. Let your neck and shoulders droop.
2. Breathe in slowly.
3. Purse your lips as though you were going to whistle, and blow out very slowly and evenly. Take twice as long to breathe out as you did to breathe in.
4. Check your relaxation. Repeat five times. If you get dizzy, rest for a few breaths.

See also the roll breathing exercise on page 300.

* Adapted from American Lung Association

Asthma - continued

○ Increase the capacity of your lungs and heart through general aerobic exercise. However, if vigorous exercise triggers asthma attacks, talk with your doctor. By adjusting your medication and your exercise routine, you and your doctor can determine a fitness program that works for you.

• Consider the use of anti-inflammatory medications to reduce the swelling of the airways. Talk with your doctor.

Home Treatment

If you can't prevent an asthma attack, the next best thing is to know when it is coming. Learn to use a peak flow meter, a device that monitors your ability to exhale. A peak flow meter can measure your progress as your prevention efforts improve your ability to breathe.

Once an asthma attack begins, good home treatment can still provide relief:

• Learn to properly use a "metered-dose inhaler." Inhalers get the right amount of medication to the airway. However, it takes some skill to use the inhaler correctly. Ask your physician to watch you use your inhaler and make suggestions for improved use.

• Drink extra fluids to thin the bronchial mucus. Try to drink at least two quarts of water per day.

• Practice the relaxation exercises on pages 300-304.

• Continue with all preventive activities discussed above.

How to Use an Inhaler

1. Shake the inhaler well. Hold the inhaler upright with your thumb on the bottom and your index and middle fingers on top.

2. Take one normal breath, then stop for a moment. Do not try to force all the air out of your lungs.

3. Close your mouth around the mouthpiece of the inhaler.

4. Squeeze the inhaler as you breathe in slowly. Continue inhaling for five to seven seconds after you have finished squeezing.

5. Remove the inhaler from your mouth, and press your lips together for about 10 seconds, then exhale through your nose.

6. Breathe normally about four or five times before taking a second dose, if needed. Repeat from step one.

Do not use an inhaler unless it has been prescribed for you by a physician.

- Take control of the asthma attack. Keep a record of what triggers attacks and what helps end them. Be confident that your home treatment will control the severity of the attack.

- If you use a humidifier, clean it thoroughly once a week.

- Get information on managing asthma. Contact the National Asthma Center, 1400 Jackson St., Denver, Colorado 80206, (800)222-5864. Also call your local chapter of the American Lung Association for additional asthma self-management publications. See Resources I1-2 on page 350.

When to Call a Health Professional

- If acute asthma symptoms have occurred for the first time.

- If asthma symptoms fail to respond promptly to treatment.

- If the attack is severe or prolonged.

- If sputum becomes discolored, particularly green, yellow, or bloody. This may be a sign of secondary bacterial infection.

- If a person with asthma, or other family members, have not been educated about immediate treatment, or if the medication required for treatment is not immediately at hand.

- To discuss exactly what to do when an attack begins. Once someone with asthma develops a good understanding of and confidence in his asthma medication, he can often handle acute episodes without immediate professional help.

- To discuss adjustments in medication. Your doctor needs your feedback to figure out the best medicine and the right dose for you.

- To discuss allergy hyposensitization shots, which may be helpful in preventing asthma attacks.

- To get a referral to a support group. Talking with others who have the same problem can be an effective way to gain confidence in dealing with prevention and treatment.

Bacterial Infections

Upper respiratory infections caused by bacteria are often hard to distinguish from those caused by a virus. Bacteria will sometimes attack the already weakened system of a person with a cold or flu. Thus, bacterial infections sometimes follow viral infections.

Older adults need to be most concerned about the development of pneumonia or bronchitis as a complication of a viral upper respiratory

Bacterial Infections - continued

infection. Other common complications include ear infections and strep throat.

You cannot prevent complications of a viral infection by taking antibiotics; antibiotics are only effective against bacterial infections. Most doctors will not prescribe antibiotics until a bacterial infection is confirmed. For important information about antibiotics, see page 337.

Viral or Bacterial?

Viral Infections

- Usually involve different parts of the body: sore throat, runny nose, headaches, muscle aches. In the abdominal area, viruses cause nausea and/or diarrhea.

- Typical viral infections: cold, flu, stomach flu.

- Antibiotics do not help.

Bacterial infections

- Bacterial infections may follow a viral infection that does not improve.

- Usually localized at a single point in the body.

- Typical bacterial infections: strep throat, ear infections.

- Antibiotics do help.

When to Call a Health Professional

- If there is a fever of 101° or higher that comes with any illness, or a fever higher than 100° that lasts more than three days.

- If the person is not starting to improve after four days.

- If sputum or nasal discharge turns from white or clear to yellow, green, or rusty-colored.

- If a cough lingers after a cold for more than 7 to 10 days without improvement.

- If there is shortness of breath.

- If there is a change in mental status. See page 138.

Bronchitis

Bronchitis is an inflammation of the bronchial tubes in the lungs. It is caused by bacteria or a virus, exposure to tobacco smoke, or pollutants in the air. It often occurs after a cold or upper respiratory infection that does not heal completely.

Inflamed bronchial tubes secrete a sticky mucus. It becomes more and more difficult for the cilia, or hairs on the bronchi, to clear out this mucus. The cough that comes with bronchitis is the body's attempt to get rid of the sticky mucus. Other bronchitis symptoms include tired-ness, low fever, sore throat, runny nose, and sometimes, wheezing.

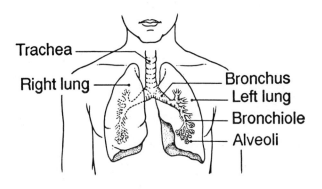

Trachea

Right lung

Bronchus
Left lung
Bronchiole
Alveoli

Lungs

Bronchitis can be serious for older adults, especially if it becomes chronic. Bronchitis is considered chronic if you have had a productive cough for more than three months per year for two years. Productive coughs produce phlegm or mucus that is expelled by coughing. A series of attacks of acute bronchitis, prolonged exposure to air pollution, or a long history of heavy smoking all contribute to chronic bronchitis.

Seventy-five percent of patients with chronic bronchitis have a history of heavy smoking.

Chronic bronchitis may occur with emphysema or chronic asthma. Any combination of these symptoms is known as chronic obstructive pulmonary disease (COPD).

Prevention

• Give proper home care to minor respiratory problems such as colds. See page 68.

• If you smoke, stop. Quitting will reduce the frequency of your cough and decrease the risk of complications.

• Avoid polluted air.

• Get a yearly flu shot. See page 22.

Get the Most Out of Your Cough

• Sit with your head bent slightly forward, feet on the floor.

• Breathe in deeply.

• Hold your breath for a few seconds.

• Cough twice, first to loosen mucus, then to bring it up.

• Breathe in by sniffing gently.

• Spit out mucus. Swallowing it can upset your stomach.

From the American Lung Association

Bronchitis - continued

Home Treatment

Self-care for bronchitis focuses on getting rid of the mucus in your lungs. Here is what you can do at home to speed healing.

- Drink 12 or more glasses of water per day. (Less, if you have congestive heart failure. See page 82.) Liquids help thin the mucus in the lungs so your cough can clear it out.

- Stop smoking. Smoke irritates the lungs and slows healing.

- Breathe moist air from a humidifier, hot shower or a sink filled with hot water. The heat and moisture will liquify mucus and help the cough bring it up.

- Twice daily, for one minute each time, lie on your stomach and hang your head and chest over the side of the bed. This helps drain the mucus. Any posture that gets the head lower than the chest will work.

- Practice pursed-lip breathing every day. See page 59.

- Have someone massage your chest and back muscles. The massage increases blood flow to the chest and helps to relax you.

When to Call a Health Professional

- If sputum that is usually clear or white turns green, rusty-brown, or yellow. This can indicate bacterial infection and requires antibiotic treatment.

- If there is difficulty in breathing, even when not coughing.

- If there is wheezing or shortness of breath.

- If any cough weakens or exhausts a person who is frail.

- If a cough lasts longer than 7 to 10 days without improvement.

Chest Pain

Call 911 or your local emergency number immediately if chest pain is severe or accompanied by shortness of breath or irregular pulse. Sweating, nausea, dizziness, and weakness may also be present. These are signs of a heart attack.

See page 84 for information.

To some people, any chest pain means "Heart Attack!" Although chest pain is the foremost warning sign of a heart attack, it is also a symptom of many other ailments. See the Chest Pain Symptom Guide on page 67.

Chest pain that increases when you press your finger on the ache signals chest-wall pain. This can be caused by strained muscles and ligaments, or inflamed cartilage in the chest wall. This is also known as costochondritis or Tietze's syndrome. Chest wall pain usually lasts only a few days. Aspirin or ibuprofen may help.

A shooting pain that lasts only a few seconds is common; there is no need for concern. Also, a quick pain at the end of a deep breath is not usually a cause for worry.

Some ulcers can cause chest pain. Ulcer-caused chest pain is worse on an empty stomach. Gallbladder pain often becomes worse after a meal. Pain that throbs with each heartbeat may be caused by an inflammation of the outside covering of the heart (pericarditis). Check out these pains with a doctor.

Three types of non-heart attack chest pain are of special concern to older adults: angina, pleurisy, and shingles.

Angina is caused by restricted circulation to the heart muscle. The symptoms are a feeling of tightness, pain, or pressure under the breastbone or across the top of the chest. Sometimes the pain spreads to the arms or jaw.

Angina is brought on by situations that stress the heart: physical exertion, a big meal, or sudden emotional upset. The average attack lasts between a few minutes and a half-hour.

Rest usually brings relief. For more information on angina, see page 85.

Pleurisy is an inflammation of the pleura, the outside covering of the lungs and lining of the chest cavity.

Pleurisy is commonly brought on by pneumonia, a broken rib, or anything that damages the chest. The pain is usually sharp and is felt along the chest wall. It will feel knife-like and stabbing after a deep breath or cough; heart pain will not. The pain from pleurisy will last until the underlying problem is cleared.

Shingles are caused by the same virus that causes chicken pox. When the virus is reactivated in the body, it often attacks the large nerves that spread from the spine around to the chest. Symptoms include a sharp, burning, or tingling pain that feels like tight bands around one side of the chest.

The pain may be followed within a few days by uncomfortable red blisters that appear at the site of the pain. The rash and the chest pain may last for 2 to 4 weeks, and sometimes months. See page 192.

Prevention

- Keep your heart healthy. See the chapters on fitness, nutrition, and stress management in this book. Anyone with diagnosed heart disease should first work with his or her physician to create a home management plan.

Chest Pain - continued

- If you live with someone who has heart problems, learn CPR (cardiopulmonary resuscitation). Call your local Red Cross, YMCA, or American Heart Association for information about training.

Home Treatment

- For chest-wall pain caused by strained muscles and ligaments:

  - Use pain relievers such as aspirin or acetaminophen.

  - Ben-Gay or Vicks VapoRub may soothe sore muscles.

  - Rest.

When to Call a Health Professional

- **CALL 911 or local emergency services IMMEDIATELY if chest pain is severe or is accompanied by:**

  - Sweating

  - Difficulty breathing

  - Nausea or vomiting

  - Dizziness

  - Irregular pulse

  - Pain that radiates to the arm, neck, or jaw

  - Increasing intensity

- If chest pain occurs in someone with a history of heart attacks, blood clots in the lung, or other chest-related illnesses.

- If chest pain is constant and nagging and is not relieved by a change in position.

- If chest pain lasts longer than two days without improvement.

Consumer Tips on Chest Pain

- Stay calm. Three times out of four, hospital chest pain evaluations show no sign of heart attack. Practice deep breathing and relaxation. See page 300.

- At the hospital expect some questions followed by an ECG (electrocardiogram). Practice the relaxation exercises on page 303 before the testing begins.

- Your doctor may suggest an angiogram or other test. Review "Get More Out of Fewer Medical Tests" on page 10.

- Always ask for a second opinion before agreeing to coronary bypass surgery. Alternatives may be available. See page 13.

Chest Pain Symptom Guide

Primary Symptom	Other Symptoms	Possible Ailment	Page #
Chest pain	Dizziness, nausea, sweating, weakness, irregular pulse	Heart attack	84
Shortness of breath	Dizziness, nausea, sweating, weakness	Heart attack	84
	Chronic cough, wheezing, colored sputum	Lung cancer Emphysema Bronchitis Pneumonia	72 70 62 73
Breastbone pain	Tightness, jaw or arm pain, increases with exercise	Angina	65
	Burning pain after eating or taking medications	Indigestion	107
	Pain increases when pressure is applied	Costochondritis	65
Chest wall pain	Recent fall, blow, or exertion	Muscle strain/rib injury	65
Sharp, burning pain	One side of chest, rash after several days	Shingles	192
Shooting pain	Worse on empty stomach	Ulcer	111
	Worse after a meal	Gallbladder	105
Stabbing pain	After deep breath or cough	Pleurisy Pneumonia	65 73
Throbbing pain	Pain with each heartbeat	Pericarditis	65

Colds

The common cold is brought to you by any one of 200 viruses. The symptoms of a cold are runny nose, red eyes, sneezing, sore throat, dry coughing, headache, and general body aches. As a cold progresses, nasal mucus may thicken. This is the stage just before a cold dries up. A cold usually lasts about one week in an adult. There is a gradual one or two day onset.

Using a mouthwash will not prevent a cold and antibiotics will not cure one. In fact, there is no cure for the common cold. If you do catch one, treat the symptoms.

Sometimes a cold will lead to more serious complications. Frail or weakened older adults need to take extra care that their colds do not progress into pneumonia, bronchitis, or an ear infection.

Prevention

- Eat well and get plenty of sleep and exercise to keep up your resistance.

- Wash your hands often, particularly when you are around people who have colds.

- Keep your hands away from your nose, eyes, and mouth.

- Use disposable tissues, not hand-kerchiefs, to reduce the spread of the virus to others.

- Humidify the bedroom or the whole house if possible.

- Don't smoke.

Home Treatment

The purpose of home treatment of a cold is to relieve symptoms and prevent complications.

- Get extra rest. Slow down just a little from your usual routine. Don't expose others.

- Drink plenty of liquids. Hot water, herbal tea, or chicken soup will help relieve congestion.

- Take aspirin or acetaminophen (Tylenol) to reduce fever and relieve aches and pain. See page 336 for precautions.

- Humidify the bedroom and take hot showers to ease nasal stuffiness.

- Watch the back of your throat for postnasal drip. If streaks of mucus appear, gargle them away to prevent a sore throat.

- Avoid "shotgun" remedies that combine drugs to treat many different symptoms. Treat each symptom separately. Take a cough medicine for a cough, a decongestant for stuffiness. See pages 334 and 335 for simple remedies you can make at home.

- Avoid antihistamines. Recent studies have found that they are not an effective treatment for colds.

- Avoid decongestants (unless approved by your physician) if you have high blood pressure or heart disease. Some decongestants are also harmful to those with thyroid disease, glaucoma, urinary problems, enlarged prostate, or diabetes. See page 334.

- Use nasal decongestant sprays for only three days or less. Continued use may lead to a "rebound effect" where the mucous membranes swell up more than before using the spray. See page 334 for nose drops you can make at home.

- Antibiotics will not help a cold.

When to Call a Health Professional

- If fever is 101° or higher.

- If there is breathing difficulty or wheezing.

- If throat is very sore, bright red, or spotted with white pus.

- If there is a foul odor from the throat, nose, or ears.

- If nasal discharge is brownish or green.

- If a cough lasts more than 7 to 10 days after a cold without improving.

- If an earache lasts more than one hour and is more than just a "stuffy" feeling.

- If the patient does not seem to be improving, or if you are quite concerned.

Coughs

Coughing is the body's way of removing foreign material or mucus from the lungs. All coughs have distinctive traits you can learn to recognize. Productive coughs produce phlegm or mucus that comes up with the cough. This kind of cough generally should not be suppressed; it is needed to clear mucus from the lungs.

Non-productive coughs are "dry" coughs that do not produce mucus. A dry or hacking cough may develop toward the end of a cold or after exposure to an irritant, such as dust or smoke.

Prevention

- If you are a smoker, quit or cut back. A dry, hacking "smoker's cough" signals that your lungs are constantly irritated.

- Drink 8 to 10 glasses of water a day. (Less if you have congestive heart failure. See page 82.)

Coughs - continued

Home Treatment

- Drink lots of water. Water helps to loosen phlegm and soothe an irritated throat. Dry, hacking coughs respond to honey in hot water, tea, or lemon juice.

- Cough drops can soothe irritated throats. Most have no effect on the cough-producing mechanism. Expensive medicine-flavored cough drops are not any better than inexpensive candy-flavored ones or hard candy.

- For coughs brought on by inhaled irritants--smoke, dust, or other pollutants--avoid exposure or wear a face mask.

- Coughs that follow viral illnesses may last up to ten days and often get worse at night. Elevate your head at night with extra pillows.

- Use an over-the-counter cough suppressant containing dextromethorphan to help quiet a dry, hacking cough so that you can sleep. Avoid dextromethorphan if you have a productive cough.

- See Cough Preparations on page 334.

When to Call a Health Professional

- If mucus becomes thick, green, or brown.

- If blood is coughed up or if the sputum becomes red-brown in color.

- If the cough involves wheezing, shortness of breath, or difficulty in breathing.

- If the cough is accompanied by a fever of 101° or higher.

- If the cough lasts longer than 7 to 10 days without improvement.

Emphysema

Emphysema is a chronic lung condition caused by repeated irritation or infection of the lung tissues. Over time, the air sacs in the lungs become permanently damaged and can no longer add oxygen to the blood or remove carbon dioxide. Emphysema is much more common in people who have been heavy smokers for a long time.

The primary symptom of emphysema is shortness of breath, especially on exertion, that worsens over time. Other symptoms can include fatigue, weight loss, frequent colds and bronchitis, and wheezing. A mild productive cough may also be present.

Together with chronic bronchitis (see page 62), emphysema contributes to the condition known as chronic obstructive pulmonary disease (COPD).

Emphysema must be diagnosed by a health professional. Once diagnosed, a detailed routine will be prescribed. There is no cure for emphysema, but proper treatment will help you lead a more normal life.

Prevention

- Don't smoke. The major cause of COPD and emphysema is cigarette smoking. See page 76.

- Stay indoors during air pollution alerts.

- Avoid people with colds or flu. Annual vaccinations against flu and a one-time pneumococcal vaccine may help. See page 22.

Home Treatment

Self-care for emphysema and COPD focuses primarily on keeping your airways clear.

- Drink lots of water--at least 8 to 10 glasses a day to keep mucus thin and fluid.

- Get the most from your cough. See page 63.

- Practice pursed-lip breathing exercises every day. See page 59.

- Exercise. General fitness can help you improve your lung function.

When to Call a Health Professional

- If you have a sudden or dramatic increase in the following symptoms:

  ○ Shortness of breath

  ○ Productive cough with green, yellow, or rusty-colored sputum

  ○ Any change in the color or texture of sputum

  ○ Wheezing

- To arrange for flu and pneumococcal vaccines.

- To arrange for a special exercise program.

- If you are a smoker and want help quitting. See page 76.

Influenza (Flu)

Influenza, or flu, is a viral illness that commonly occurs in the winter. It usually affects many people at once. (The name "influenza" comes from the Italian word for "influence.")

Influenza has symptoms similar to a cold, but they are usually more severe and come on quite suddenly.

The flu is commonly thought of as a respiratory illness, but the whole body can be affected. Symptoms include weakness, fatigue, muscle

Influenza - continued

aches, headaches, fever (101° to 102°), chills, sneezing, and runny nose. Symptoms may last five to seven days.

Flu can be dangerous for older adults, especially those who are already weakened by another illness. High-risk conditions include:

- Age 65 or older and frail
- Chronic lung diseases
- Heart disease
- Diabetes or other metabolic disorders
- Anemia
- Illness or treatments that weaken the immune system

Those in the high risk groups are in greatest danger from flu and its complications, which include bacterial pneumonia, bronchitis, and sinus and ear infections.

Prevention

- Get a flu shot each autumn if you are over 65, or if you have any of the conditions listed above. For more on flu shots, see page 22.

- Keep up your resistance to infection with a good diet, plenty of rest, and regular exercise.

- Avoid exposure to the virus. Wash your hands often and keep your hands away from your nose, eyes, and mouth.

Home Treatment

- Get plenty of bed rest.

- Drink extra fluids, at least one full glass of water or juice every hour.

- Take acetaminophen (Tylenol) to relieve head and muscle aches.

When to Call a Health Professional

- If you are in a high-risk group. See above.

- If cough brings up heavy thick mucus.

- If there is a fever of 101° or higher.

- If a patient seems to get better, then gets worse again.

- If flu-like symptoms or a red rash occur ten days to three weeks after a possible tick bite. This may indicate Lyme disease, a bacterial infection spread by deer ticks.

Lung Cancer

Lung cancer is the number one cancer killer of men and women. It is most often found in long-term smokers over age 50. In all cancers, abnormal cells or cancer cells crowd out and destroy normal, healthy tissue. Lung cells can become cancerous when repeatedly damaged by smoke, chemicals, or other irritants that are inhaled.

Secondhand tobacco smoke, radon, and asbestos dust can also contribute to lung cancer. A combination of risk factors, such as a smoker whose work involves handling asbestos, greatly increases the chance of getting lung cancer.

The symptoms of lung cancer are very similar to other chest and lung problems: chronic cough, shortness of breath, wheezing, repeated lung infections or pneumonia, pain in the chest wall, or spitting up pus-filled or bloody sputum.

The kind of symptom will depend upon where in the lung the cancerous cells are found. There may be no symptoms in the early stages, making lung cancer difficult to detect. Any chronic respiratory symptom in a smoker should be checked out by a doctor.

Prevention

- If you smoke, quit. Ten to fifteen years after quitting, an exsmoker's risk of cancer is about the same as a nonsmoker's. You don't have to wait that long for benefits; lungs begin to heal almost immediately after quitting. See page 76.

- Avoid secondhand smoke. Even if you have never smoked, breathing in others' smoke puts you at risk.

- Test your home for radon. There are several testing kits available.

Call your local American Lung Association chapter for information.

Home Treatment

- See "Winning Over Serious Illness" on page 311.

When to Call a Health Professional

- If chest pain lasts longer than two days.

- If a cough lasts longer than 7 to 10 days without improvement.

- If there are several bouts of pneumonia in a year.

- If blood is coughed up or if sputum becomes red-brown in color.

- If there is wheezing, shortness of breath, or difficulty in breathing,

- If there is fever of 101° or higher.

- If lung cancer has been diagnosed. Any cancer requires continual physician supervision.

Pneumonia

Pneumonia is an infection or inflammation of the alveoli, the smallest air passages in the lungs. These passages fill up with pus or mucus, preventing oxygen from reaching the blood.

Pneumonia - continued

Pneumonia is a serious problem for older adults whose resistance is poor. It is the fifth leading cause of death among people over age 65.

Pneumonia often follows or accompanies a cold, flu, or bronchitis. Look for fever and for a cough that brings up greenish-yellow or reddish-brown sputum. There may be pain in the chest, especially when coughing or taking a deep breath. Breathing itself may be labored or rapid. Sweating, weakness, loss of appetite, and stomach discomfort may also be present. As the body is deprived of oxygen, the lips and nails may turn bluish in color (cyanosis).

Prevention

- Maintain the body's normal resistance with good diet, rest, and exercise.

- Take care of minor illnesses. Don't try to "tough" your way through them. See home treatment for colds on page 68.

- Get a pneumococcal immunization. This is generally recommended for people over age 65 and for anyone with chronic heart and lung illnesses or diabetes. The immunization should be given only once.

- Avoid smoke and other irritants.

Home Treatment

- Call a health professional if you suspect pneumonia. After the diagnosis is given, follow the home treatment below.

  - Drink lots of water--at least 8 to 10 glasses a day. Extra fluids are necessary to help thin mucus.

  - Get lots of rest. Don't try to rush recovery.

When to Call a Health Professional

- If, during any respiratory illness, there is rapid or labored breathing.

- If a cough following a cold lasts longer than 7 to 10 days without improving.

- If there is a fever of 101° or higher.

- If an unexplained cough appears a few weeks after a cold.

- If there is a productive cough with green, yellow, or rusty-colored sputum.

- To arrange for a pneumococcal immunization.

Sinusitis

Sinusitis is an infection of the sinuses. The sinuses are cavities, or hollow spaces, in the head which are lined with mucous membranes.

These cavities usually drain easily unless there is an inflammation or infection. Sinusitis may follow a head cold and is often associated with hay fever or asthma. There are two categories of sinusitis: acute, lasting less than three weeks; and chronic, lasting longer.

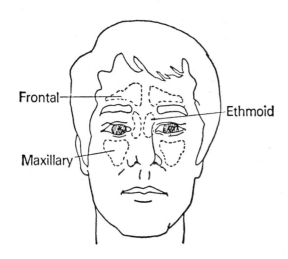

Sinus Cavities

The key symptom of sinusitis is pain in the forehead, under the eyes, or opposite the bridge of the nose. There may also be headache, fever (if the sinuses are infected), runny nose, postnasal drip (mucus running down the throat), sore throat, and pain in the upper teeth. Headaches caused by sinusitis may occur on rising and get worse in the afternoon or when bending over.

Prevention

- Treat colds promptly. Blow your nose gently and with your mouth open to avoid forcing mucus into a sinus.

- Stop smoking. Smokers are more prone to sinusitis than nonsmokers.

Home Treatment

- When you first notice sinus pain, lie down on your back and apply alternating hot and cold compresses to your forehead and cheeks, about one minute each, for ten minutes. If needed, repeat four times daily, giving the last treatment at bedtime. This treatment seems to stimulate the flow of mucus.

- Apply decongestant nose drops to each nostril while lying down. See page 334 for types of decongestants. Do not use decongestant nose drops for more than three days.

- Watch the back of your throat for postnasal drip. If streaks of mucus appear, gargle with warm water to prevent a sore throat.

- Increase home humidity, especially in bedrooms.

- Drink extra fluids to keep mucus thin. Drink a glass of water or juice every waking hour.

Sinusitis - continued

- Breathe moist air from a humidifier, hot shower, or sink filled with hot water.

- Take aspirin or acetaminophen for headache.

When to Call a Health Professional

- If you feel pain and tenderness along the ridge between the nose and lower eyelid.

- If there is fever of 101° or higher.

- If there is increased swelling of the face.

- If severe headache pain is not eased by aspirin or acetaminophen.

- If there is bleeding from the nose.

- If there is increased thick brownish-green nasal discharge.

- If there are changes or blurring in vision.

- If there is no improvement after two days of home treatment.

Quitting Smoking

If you have been smoking for 30 to 40 years, you may think it's too late to quit. It's never too late. Here's the good news:

- Your risk of heart disease begins to drop almost immediately, and after 10 years it is close to that of a nonsmoker.

- Your lungs begin to heal immediately, and after 10 to 15 years, your risk of lung cancer drops to nearly that of a nonsmoker.

- Your circulation will improve, increasing the amount of blood that reaches your brain. This is important in helping you stay mentally strong, and in reducing your risk of stroke.

Quitting smoking is the most important thing you can do for your own health and the health of those around you. However, it won't be easy. Chances are you have already tried once or twice. As Mark Twain once said, "Quitting smoking is the easiest thing I have ever done. I've done it a hundred times."

No one can tell you when or how to quit smoking. Only you know why you smoke and what will be most difficult as you try to stop. The important thing is that you try. Believe that you will succeed, if not the first time, then the second time, or twenty-second time.

Tips for Quitting

Preparation

- Decide for yourself how and when you will quit. About half of ex-smokers quit "cold turkey"; the other half cut down gradually.

Ten Good Reasons to Quit at Age 50 or Better

1. Your body will begin to heal itself.
2. Shortness of breath and cough decrease.
3. Stamina and energy are improved.
4. Fewer colds and illnesses.
5. You'll smell good.
6. Taste buds and sense of smell come back to life.
7. More spending money.
8. It's good for loved ones.
9. Be in control of your life.
10. It's a good idea.

- Figure out why you smoke. Do you smoke to pep yourself up? To relax? Do you like the ritual of smoking? Do you smoke to deal with negative feelings? Do you smoke out of habit, often without realizing what you're doing?

  The key is to cultivate a healthful alternative that accomplishes for you what smoking does. For example, if you like to have something to do with your hands, pick up something else: coin, worry beads, pen or pencil. If you like to have something in your mouth, substitute sugarless gum or minted toothpicks.

- List your reasons for quitting. Keep reminding yourself of your goal.

- Replace your pleasures. Plan a regular, healthful reward that you will experience because you have quit smoking. Take the money you save by not buying cigarettes and spend it on yourself.

- Think of yourself as an exsmoker. Think positive.

Action

- Set a quit date and stick to it. Choose a time that will be busy but not stressful.

- Remember the word HALT and try to avoid becoming too Hungry, Angry, Lonely, or Tired. These are situations that make many people want to smoke. Alcohol is another trigger for many smokers; try to avoid it, too.

- Change your surroundings. Remove ashtrays and all reminders of smoking. Choose non-smoking sections in restaurants. Do things that are incompatible with smoking, like taking a walk or going to a concert.

- Ask for help and support. Choose a trusted friend, preferably another exsmoker, to give you a helping hand over the rough spots.

- Set up rewards for yourself.

- Good books with good information can help. See Resource W1 on page 352.

Quitting Smoking - continued

- Choose a reliable smoking cessation program to help you get started. The key question is, "What is your success rate at the end of one year?" Good programs have at least a 20 percent success rate; great programs have a 50 percent success rate. Programs that claim higher numbers may be too good to be true.

- Know what to expect. Physical withdrawal symptoms may last one to three weeks, but the worst will be over in just a few days. After that, it is all psychological. Prepare yourself for some irritability. Counter with relaxation. See Chapter 21.

- Drink lots of water and other healthful liquids to help flush the nicotine out of your system. Keep alcohol to a bare minimum, if any.

- Watch your diet. Your appetite will perk up, so have low-calorie snacks available. Carrot and celery sticks are particularly good.

- Get out and exercise. It will distract you, keep off unwanted pounds, and release tension.

- Be prepared for slip-ups. If you do, forgive yourself and learn from the experience. Remember that you will not fail as long as you keep trying.

- Good luck!

If your heart has peace, nothing can disturb you.
The Dalai Lama

5

Heart and Circulation Problems

Your heart and circulatory system feed and nurture every cell in your body. To a great extent, they determine how far you can walk, how late you can dance, and how long you can garden. The heart is the key to a physically robust life at any age, but especially as you get older.

Disorders of the heart and circulatory system kill more people than all other causes combined. Major risk factors include:

- Smoking

- High blood pressure

- Obesity

- Cholesterol over 240

- Family history

This chapter highlights the problems that can occur with the heart and circulatory system and what you can do to prevent these problems.

Your Largest Muscles

The heart and circulatory system are muscles. The circulatory system is a long (12,400 miles) tubular muscle that carries blood from your heart, through arteries, to the farthest reaches of your body and back to your heart through veins. Your heart is also a hollow muscle. When it contracts, it forces the blood in it to surge out through the arteries. When these muscles are well-conditioned, they expand and relax easily. When they are out of shape, they stiffen and lose their flexibility.

Muscles need oxygen in order to work. Without oxygen, a muscle soon begins to die. When a part of the heart muscle dies, it is called a heart attack, or myocardial infarction.

Reduced blood supply to the heart causes most heart attacks. Blood supply is reduced as a result of atherosclerosis in the coronary arteries.

Atherosclerosis

Atherosclerosis is the gradual build-up of fatty deposits inside the arteries. Atherosclerosis occurs in a three-step process:

1. The strong contractions of the heart and the pressure of the blood it pumps cause tiny tears on the inside of the arteries. High blood pressure increases the tearing.

2. Fat and cholesterol in the blood stick to these tiny tears. Over time, the cholesterol calcifies and hardens into plaques (sometimes called "hardening of the arteries").

3. These plaques narrow the arteries and reduce the blood supply to the heart muscle and other parts of the body.

When atherosclerosis occurs in the large arteries that supply blood to the heart muscle, it is known as coronary artery disease. The plaques in the coronary arteries can interfere with or block the flow of blood to the heart muscle. When the heart doesn't get enough blood, it can no longer work properly.

The term "heart disease" is often used to refer to coronary artery disease, or to a number of other conditions that it can cause. Angina (page 65), congestive heart failure (page 82), and heart attack (page 84) are all conditions that can result from coronary artery disease.

When atherosclerosis blocks blood flow to the brain, transient ischemic attacks (TIAs) (page 93) and strokes (page 92) can occur.

A form of dementia, called multi-infarct dementia, is the result of plaque formation in the small arteries of the brain (page 143).

Atherosclerosis can also affect the arteries in the legs, causing a condition called peripheral vascular disease (page 89).

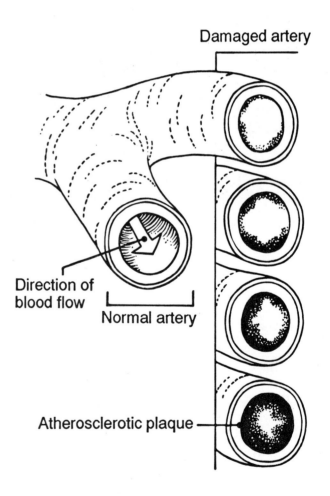

Damaged artery

Direction of blood flow

Normal artery

Atherosclerotic plaque

Atherosclerosis

Prevention

Fortunately, the diseases and disabilities caused by atherosclerosis are among the most preventable of all major illnesses. Three simple measures will help prevent atherosclerosis:

- Control blood pressure to reduce arterial tears.

- Reduce cholesterol and triglycerides in the blood.

- Exercise to keep arteries strong and flexible.

Control blood pressure to reduce arterial tears.

- Avoid nicotine. It constricts your arteries, raises blood pressure, increases arterial tearing, speeds atherosclerosis, and reduces the oxygen level in the blood.

- Maintain a healthy body weight. Excess body fat increases blood pressure and adds stress to the heart and circulatory system.

- Become more aware of your anger, anxiety, and fear. These emotions trigger the release of adrenaline and increase blood pressure. These are normal human feelings, but if they are a big part of your day, start using stress management techniques (pages 300 to 304).

- Avoid illegal drugs, especially cocaine; and amphetamines. These constrict the arteries and increase the workload of the heart.

- Follow the guidelines for controlling blood pressure on page 86.

Reduce cholesterol in the bloodstream.

- Decrease the amount of cholesterol and saturated fat you eat. You can reverse atherosclerosis by limiting the number of calories of fat you eat to 10 percent of your total calories. For most people, even dropping to a 25 percent fat diet would make a big difference. See page 285.

- Reduce adrenaline, which not only increases your blood pressure, but also tells your body to hold onto the fats it would ordinarily excrete. You can reduce adrenaline in three ways:

  - Stop smoking.

  - Learn to recognize and deal with anger, anxiety, and fear.

  - Avoid cocaine, speed, and other illicit drugs.

- Maintain ideal weight. The more fat in your diet, the more fat in your blood.

- Control diabetes. Uncontrolled blood sugar levels increase the amount of fat in the blood.

Atherosclerosis - continued

Exercise to keep arteries strong and flexible.

- Add aerobic exercise to your daily routine. Exercise keeps your arteries and heart flexible and strong. In addition, aerobic exercise fights atherosclerosis by:

  - Lowering cholesterol levels

  - Reducing blood pressure

  - Keeping weight down

  - Boosting relaxation and well-being.

Walking, swimming, jogging, biking, hiking, and dancing are all good aerobic exercises. See page 262.

Congestive Heart Failure

The heart doesn't completely fail in congestive heart failure (CHF). When the heart has been damaged by heart disease, long-term high blood pressure, or a heart attack, it can no longer pump effectively. This is called congestive heart failure. The kidneys respond to the reduced circulation by retaining salt and water in the body, which further strains the heart.

The left side of the heart pumps blood containing oxygen from the lungs to the cells of your body. When your body has used the oxygen in the blood, it returns to the heart. The right side of the heart then pumps the blood to the lungs, where it gets a fresh load of oxygen. This process goes on every minute of every day of your life.

When the left side of the heart is damaged, the heart is unable to pump all the blood that is returning to it from the lungs. This is called left-sided CHF. The blood backs up in the lungs and causes the following symptoms:

- Shortness of breath and wheezing, even while at rest

- Difficulty breathing when lying down

- Sleep disturbances; waking up panting or with a feeling of suffocation

- A dry, hacking, non-productive cough when lying down, that is relieved by sitting up

- Fatigue and lethargy

When the right side of the heart is damaged, the heart is unable to pump all the blood returning to it from the body. This is called right-sided CHF. The blood backs up into the legs and the liver, causing the following symptoms:

- Swollen feet and ankles (edema)

- Swollen neck veins

- Constant pain just below the ribs on the right side (from an enlarged liver)

- Fatigue and lethargy

Prevention

Follow the guidelines for prevention of atherosclerosis on page 81. Taking these steps will help prevent most causes of heart failure.

Home Treatment

Work with your doctor to develop a program of diet, rest, and medication that will help you to manage congestive heart failure. Some general guidelines include:

- Stop smoking.

- Cut back on salt to limit water retention.

- Drink less fluid if edema is present. However, do not drink less than five 8-ounce cups per day.

- Avoid alcoholic beverages and those containing caffeine.

- Elevate swollen feet and ankles above the level of your heart with pillows.

- Review all prescription and over-the-counter drugs that you take with your doctor. Some medications make your body retain more fluid, further straining your heart.

- Sleep propped up on pillows or in a comfortable chair to make breathing easier at night.

- Avoid exercise that causes you to breathe hard or become very short of breath. Stretching and walking at a moderate pace are often fine. Ask your doctor about an appropriate exercise level.

When to Call a Health Professional

- To confirm the diagnosis and establish a treatment plan.

- To work with your doctor to develop a safe and realistic exercise schedule.

- If swelling increases in your legs at night.

- To ask about medications you may be taking that increase salt retention.

- Get immediate medical attention for:

  - Severe shortness of breath

  - Foamy, pink mucus with your cough

  - Sweating and pale color

  - Chest pain not relieved by rest or medication

Heart Attack

A heart attack happens when part of the heart muscle dies because of too little oxygen. This is also called a myocardial (heart muscle) infarction (tissue death), or M.I.

When blood flows through an artery of the heart that has been narrowed by atherosclerosis, it slows down, becomes turbulent, and tends to clot. When a clot forms, blood is cut off from the portion of the heart muscle below the clot. Once the blood supply is cut off, the affected muscle begins to die.

M.I.s can also occur when the rhythm of the heartbeat becomes very irregular (arrhythmia). If the arrhythmia is severe, it will prevent sufficient blood from getting to the heart muscle. That may cause the affected area of the heart muscle to die.

The size and location of the M.I. determines how the heart will continue to function. If only a small amount of heart muscle dies, the victim may recover quickly. If the muscle death is extensive, there is less chance of recovery.

Any or all of these symptoms may precede or follow a heart attack:

- Chest pain
  - Often a crushing or squeezing pain or a feeling of tightness.
  - The pain can radiate to the arms, elbows, shoulder, back, neck, jaw, or top of stomach.

- Difficulty breathing; shortness of breath

- Sweating

- Rapid or irregular pulse

- Nausea, vomiting

- Confusion

- Loss of consciousness

CPR Training

Cardiopulmonary resuscitation (CPR) can save lives and improve recovery from heart attacks. Consider signing up for a CPR class or taking a refresher course. They are offered through the American Red Cross, the American Heart Association, and other community groups.

If you have taken a CPR course, the following will refresh your memory:
1. Check consciousness.
2. Check breathing.
3. Open airway.
4. Rescue breathing (2 breaths).
5. Check pulse.
6. If no pulse, begin CPR; 15 compressions, then 2 breaths.
7. Continue until help arrives.

Note: Older adults and people with diabetes may not experience chest pain or other symptoms during a heart attack. These "silent" heart attacks can be detected only by an electrocardiogram (ECG).

Prevention

Follow the guidelines for preventing atherosclerosis on page 81.

Home Treatment

Time is extremely important when a person is having a heart attack. Drugs that dissolve clots and drugs that reduce the oxygen needs of the heart are most effective if given **within one hour of the onset of symptoms.**

- Have the heart attack victim lie down to reduce the strain on the heart.

- Loosen any clothing that may restrict breathing.

- Call 911 or local emergency service to request an ambulance. Remember how important the first hour is. If you live a long way from ambulance services, call the hospital for advice on whether to drive to the hospital. Never let the victim drive.

- If the victim has nitroglycerine tablets for angina, give them as prescribed.

- If the person loses consciousness and you cannot find a pulse, begin CPR and do not stop until emergency personnel take your place.

- Once you begin to recover from a heart attack, dedicate yourself to practices that will prevent a second heart attack.

Angina or Heart Attack?

Angina is caused by poor circulation to the heart muscle. It is described on page 65.

Once you are diagnosed as having angina, it helps to distinguish the difference between angina and heart attack pain:

- Angina may come on with exertion and quickly gets better with rest.

- Angina is short-term pain, lasting only a few minutes. The pain of a heart attack usually lasts an hour or more, or until relieved by medications.

- Angina is relieved by the prescribed dose of nitroglycerine. The pain of a heart attack is not.

- Angina usually is not accompanied by the heavy perspiration, shortness of breath, and nausea associated with a heart attack.

- If you are in doubt, call your doctor, 911, or your local emergency service.

Heart Attack - continued

When to Call a Health Professional

Call 911 or other emergency services immediately for severe chest pain or if:

- Chest pain is not relieved by resting or by your prescribed dose of nitroglycerine.

- Chest pain is associated with:

  - Pain radiating to arm, elbow, shoulder, back, neck, or jaw

  - Shortness of breath/difficulty breathing

  - Rapid or irregular pulse

  - Sweating

  - Nausea or vomiting

  - Dizziness and confusion

- If you have any chest pain of unknown cause that continues for 15 minutes or longer.

Note: If the chest pain is not accompanied by any of the symptoms described on the previous pages, see pages 64 and 67.

High Blood Pressure (Hypertension)

Blood pressure is a measurement of the pressure your blood exerts against the artery walls.

As your heart pumps out a load of oxygen-rich blood, the pressure in your arteries surges. The pressure drops between heart beats. The pressure when the heart contracts is called the systolic pressure (the first number in blood pressure readings). The pressure between beats, when the heart at rest, is called the diastolic pressure.

You have high blood pressure, or hypertension, if your blood pressure is 140/90 or higher. Despite what a lot of people think, high blood pressure does not make you dizzy, nervous, or tense. Most affected people have no symptoms. The only way to know for sure is to measure it regularly.

Untreated high blood pressure can lead to:

- Stroke

- Heart disease and heart attack

- Loss of vision

- Kidney failure

High blood pressure is very common; more than half of all older adults have hypertension. Those at increased risk include: African-Americans; people who smoke; those who are overweight; and those who have a family history of hypertension.

The goal of blood pressure control is to maintain a systolic pressure of less than 140 and a diastolic pressure of less than 90.

Prevention

- Know your blood pressure. If your last measurement was 140/90 or higher, check it every month. See page 347.

- Don't smoke. Nicotine constricts arteries and keeps blood pressure high.

- Gradually increase the amount of aerobic exercise in your day. See page 258.

- Maintain a good weight for you. See page 295.

- Avoid cocaine and other drugs that affect your heart.

Home Treatment

- Cut back on sodium. Salt may make your body retain fluids. The extra fluid increases your blood pressure and makes your heart work harder. See page 294 for tips on reducing sodium.

  Some guidelines recommend no more than one teaspoon per day (and that includes the salt found in processed food!).

- If you are taking medications for high blood pressure, take them regularly. Skipping doses can have adverse effects on your blood pressure.

- Make sure you're getting enough calcium and potassium in your diet. You can:

  o Drink more low-fat milk. See page 292 for more on calcium.

  o Eat a banana every day for more potassium.

- If you often feel angry or anxious, practice a relaxation technique daily. See page 300.

- Keep your alcohol consumption moderate; no more than one drink per day.

- Avoid taking antihistamines, and take decongestants only under the advice of a physician. These drugs can raise blood pressure.

- Get regular exercise. Besides lowering blood pressure, exercise will:

  o Reduce your body weight

  o Improve your self-image

  o Reduce your stress

  o Increase the sparkle in your eye

Hypertension - continued

- Learn to take your own blood pressure. Ask your pharmacist to recommend a blood pressure kit. See page 344. Your doctor or a nurse can show you how to use it.

- Quit smoking. See page 76 for tips on how to quit.

When to Call a Health Professional

- If you have had two or more blood pressure measurements with a systolic pressure over 140 and/or a diastolic pressure greater than 90.

- If you believe you are experiencing dizziness or other side effects from your medications. (See also Dizziness on page 166.) Talk with your doctor before stopping any prescribed medication.

Irregular Heartbeats (Arrhythmias)

Normally the heart beats with a regular rhythm and at a rate appropriate for the work your body is doing. Irregular heartbeats, or arrhythmias, occur when the heart beats too fast, too slow, or with an irregular rhythm. Most arrhythmias are harmless, but some can be life-threatening.

Anything that injures the heart can alter the pacing of the beats. Examples are:

Fainting Spells

A fainting spell, known medically as syncope (sin-ko-pee), is an indication that your brain is not getting enough oxygen. Syncope is often caused by heart problems, like arrhythmias, or by nervous system disorders. The signs of an approaching fainting spell are nausea, sweating, and a "graying-out" of vision.

The biggest dangers of a fainting spell are the fractures and head injuries that might result from keeling over. Lie down or sit until the symptoms pass.

You will need to consult with your doctor about any fainting spells. Also see page 166 for information on vertigo and dizziness.

- Atherosclerosis in the coronary arteries

- A heart attack

- Stretching of the heart muscle through congestive heart failure

One way you will notice a change in rhythm is by feeling a "skipped" beat, or a "flip-flop" in your chest. These are often called palpitations. You may also experience chest discomfort, shortness of breath, a feeling of lightheadedness, or even a fainting spell. When this happens, write down the time, date, what you were doing, the number of "skipped" beats per minute, and any other symptoms you experienced.

If necessary, heartbeat irregularities can be controlled by drugs or with an artificial pacemaker.

Prevention

- Avoid tobacco, caffeine, and alcohol. These contribute to episodes of arrhythmia.

- Gradually increase the amount of aerobic exercise in your day. Keeping your heart strong will reduce the frequency and severity of arrhythmias.

Home Treatment

- Learn to take your pulse and keep a written record of any instances of irregular heartbeats.

- When your heart is reacting to stress or your emotions, practice a relaxation technique. See page 300.

When to Call a Health Professional

- If you experience several "skipped" beats in a row.

- If you suddenly experience a very rapid or very slow heartbeat without an obvious cause.

- If you experience any new disturbance of heart rate or rhythm, report it to your doctor.

- Call immediately if you are also experiencing:

  o Chest pain

  o Shortness of breath

  o Nausea

  o Dizziness or fainting

  o Sweating

Peripheral Vascular Disease

Sometimes, atherosclerosis builds up in the arteries of the leg. As the fatty deposits reduce the flow of blood to the legs, leg pain results. This condition is called peripheral vascular disease.

The primary symptom of peripheral vascular disease is leg pain that occurs during walking or other exercise. This pain is called intermittent claudication (claw-di-kay-shun). The pain is sometimes described as tight or squeezing, and is relieved by rest.

Other symptoms may include occasional tingling, numbness, or coldness in the feet, loss of hair on the feet, and irregular growth of toenails.

Peripheral vascular disease will usually get worse with time. Eventually, if the blood flow becomes completely blocked, skin ulcers, infections, and gangrene can set in. Amputation may become necessary.

Vascular Disease - continued

Claudication can also occur in the hips and buttocks due to advanced atherosclerosis in those arteries.

Prevention

- Follow the prevention guidelines for atherosclerosis. See page 81. Work on getting your cholesterol down. See page 288.

- If you have diabetes, keep your blood sugar under control. See page 121.

- Control your blood pressure. See High Blood Pressure on page 86.

Home Treatment

- Stop smoking now! People who continue to smoke after developing symptoms are over ten times more likely to lose their limbs than those who quit smoking.

- Gradually increase your aerobic exercise.

  - The goal is to increase the time you can exercise before pain begins.

  - Walking, bicycling, or using a stationary bicycle are good choices.

  - Rest when pain begins.

- Reduce the fat in your diet. See page 285.

- Keep your cholesterol down. See page 288.

- Avoid extreme cold.

- Take good care of your feet. See page 122.

- Avoid socks or stockings that leave elastic band marks on your calves or legs.

When to Call a Health Professional

- If this is your first incidence of severe leg, hip, or buttock pain with exercise.

- If, despite home treatment, the pain gets worse, comes on sooner, or occurs at rest.

- If leg pain extends to the foot.

- If you notice coolness or lack of feeling in the foot of the affected limb.

- If you develop open sores on your legs or feet.

Phlebitis/ Thrombophlebitis

If a vein becomes inflamed, it is called phlebitis. If a clot forms at the site of the inflammation, it is called thrombophlebitis. However, thrombophlebitis is sometimes called phlebitis for short. It occurs most commonly in the leg veins. It can affect veins both near the skin (superficial phlebitis) and deep in the leg.

Symptoms of phlebitis include redness, swelling, and tenderness around a surface vein of the lower leg. Occasionally, you can feel a small clot on the edge of the inflammation. These symptoms are uncomfortable, but can usually be relieved by rest and anti-inflammatory drugs, such as aspirin and ibuprofen (Advil).

Thrombophlebitis in a deep leg vein is much more serious. These clots may break away from the leg vein and lodge in the lung, often with fatal consequences.

Symptoms of deep vein thrombophlebitis include:

- Increasing leg pain, especially after standing

- Swelling of one leg

- Tenderness, heat, and redness in the leg without observable cause

Risk factors for thrombophlebitis include injury, heart or lung disease, cancer, estrogen replacement therapy, and long periods of bed rest. Tight garters and sitting in one position for long periods may also cause problems.

Thrombophlebitis above the knee is treated with strong drugs to prevent further clotting. Hospital care and close monitoring may be needed to prevent complications. Clots below the knee usually do not need anti-coagulants. They result in serious problems much less often.

Prevention

- Regular exercise will increase the muscle tone of the lower legs and help prevent clots from forming.

- Contract and relax your leg muscles frequently if you stand or sit for long periods of time.

- Avoid socks or stockings that leave elastic band marks on your calves or legs.

- Get up, move, and change positions often.

- Ask your doctor about wearing strong elastic support stockings.

Home Treatment

For superficial phlebitis:

- Rest with the leg elevated, but avoid complete inactivity or staying in one position too long.

- Use aspirin or other anti-inflammatory drugs as recommended by your physician.

- Apply warm compresses to the affected area.

- Wear elastic support stockings.

Phlebitis - continued

When to Call a Health Professional

- If there is heaviness and pain in the leg.

- If you have unexplained swelling in the leg.

- If the leg is tender and warm to the touch.

Stroke

A stroke happens when a portion of the brain dies from too little oxygen. Arteries in the brain can become blocked by a clot or atherosclerosis. They can also rupture from the wear and tear of high blood pressure. If either event prevents blood and oxygen from reaching a part of the brain, a stroke results.

If the blood supply is not restored, the entire area fed by the artery will die and the person will lose the functions associated with that section of the brain.

Stroke is a serious emergency and prompt medical attention is needed. Watch for these symptoms:

- Progressive loss of speech, sight, or sensation over a period of a few minutes or hours

- Sudden weakness or loss of sensation in an arm and/or leg (usually

A Caregiver's Guide For Heart Attack and Stroke

When a life-threatening crisis like a heart attack or stroke occurs, the victim may feel vulnerable, frightened, and depressed. Fears of never working, loving, or playing again are common. Death was close, it may seem, and may come again at any minute. It is hard on loved ones, too. Caregiving can be a very painful experience.

Fortunately, there are many professionals who can help you help your patient. Rehabilitation and physical therapists can establish home activities that will speed healing. Occupational therapists can advise you on adaptive devices and home set-up to encourage independence.

Caregivers need support, too. Gather your friends around you. Talk with someone who has survived a stroke or heart attack. They will help you learn that much is possible in the rehabilitation process. The difficulties you see today may be much improved in the weeks and months ahead.

For more information, see Chapter 24, Caregiver Secrets. For information on support groups, contact your local chapter of the American Heart Association.

on the same side). One side of the face may also be affected.

- Rapid onset of double vision or slurred speech

- Sudden onset of severe headache

- Loss of consciousness

People who smoke, or who have diabetes, high blood pressure, high cholesterol levels, or heart disease are at increased risk for stroke.

A person who has experienced a transient ischemic attack (TIA) should consider it a warning sign for stroke. The symptoms are similar to a stroke: sudden weakness or numbness in a limb, and difficulties with speech and vision. However, there is a critical difference between the two. Unlike a stroke, most TIA episodes last only a few minutes and symptoms disappear within 24 hours. Even if the occurrence seems over before it has begun, a diagnosis and evaluation need to be made by a physician.

The impact of a stroke depends upon the location and extent of the damage to the brain. Stroke effects can range from sudden death to a slight slurring of speech, and include:

- Weakness or total paralysis on one side of the body

- Changes in behavior and/or emotions

- Loss of memory

- Difficulty speaking or making sense of words and pictures

- Vision loss on one side

- Depression and withdrawal

Prevention

- Control your blood pressure. This is the most important risk factor for strokes.

- Don't smoke. Women who smoke a pack a day are nearly four times more likely to have a stroke than women who don't smoke at all. Male smokers also have a high risk of stroke.

- If you have diabetes, keep your blood sugar under strict control. See page 121.

- Get regular aerobic exercise. Flexible arteries are less likely to burst. See pages 258 to 264.

- Reduce the amount of fat and cholesterol in your diet.

- If you have high blood pressure or diabetes, ask your doctor about taking one regular aspirin a day.

- Drink alcohol in moderation, no more than one drink per day. Alcohol increases the chance of having a stroke.

Stroke - continued

Home Treatment

- Know the early warning signs of a stroke and be ready to seek emergency care if they occur.

- If someone you love has had a stroke, your efforts will go to giving care that will speed healing. Start rehabilitation early and involve family members and friends. Active family involvement will help recovery. See the Caregiver's Guide on page 92, and "Winning over Serious Illness" on page 311.

When to Call a Health Professional

Consult your physician immediately if you have any of the following symptoms:

- Temporary loss of speech, or difficulty speaking or understanding speech.

- Sudden onset of dizziness or unsteadiness that is not explained by other causes.

- Temporary weakness or numbness of the face, arm, leg, or on one side of the body.

- Sudden double vision, dimmed vision, or loss of vision, particularly in one eye.

- Sudden onset of a severe headache. Also see page 129.

Varicose Veins

Varicose veins are twisted, blue, and swollen veins close to the surface of the skin. They most often occur in the legs. Other symptoms include itching, aching, swelling of the ankles, and a feeling of heaviness in the legs.

Valves in the leg veins help blood flow from the legs back to the heart. If the valves become damaged or weakened, the blood pools in the veins and causes the vein wall to swell outward.

If the veins deep in the legs are involved, complications such as swollen legs and skin ulcers around the ankles may set in.

Some people have a strong family history of varicose veins and are much more likely to develop them. Pregnant women, and those who are overweight or who spend much of their time standing are particularly at risk.

Treatment, either with injections or surgical stripping of the affected vein, is costly and usually only temporarily successful. Prevention and conservative measures to control the progress of vein damage is most successful.

Prevention

- Get regular exercise. Walking improves leg and vein strength.

- Wear elastic support stockings when standing for long periods of time.

- If you must stand for long periods of time, sit down when you can with your feet elevated above your heart. This will improve blood return.

- Maintain a good body weight. See page 295.

Home Treatment

Once the varicose veins are present, home treatment cannot make them disappear. However, practice the prevention tips above to limit the progress of vein damage.

When to Call a Health Professional

- If the vein becomes very tender, swollen, red, or warm to the touch.

- If ulcers or open sores develop on your legs or feet.

*I am living at peace with men
and at war with my innards.*
Antonio Machado

6

Digestive and Urinary Problems

Your digestive system is a hard-working food distributor. Its job is to bring useful nutrients and minerals to the body. The urinary system eliminates unnecessary and harmful products.

Usually, the digestive system is working all the time: 24 hours a day, 7 days a week, 52 weeks a year. Except for brief episodes of illness, most people find that their food distributor gives them very few problems.

With good food and drink going in, there is little to go wrong. Occasionally, however, your digestive and urinary systems encounter trouble. When they do, the guidelines in this chapter may help.

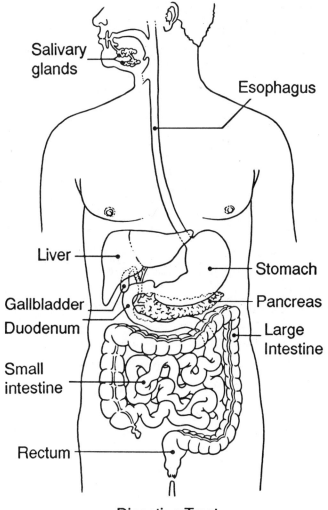

Salivary glands

Esophagus

Liver

Stomach

Gallbladder

Pancreas

Duodenum

Large Intestine

Small intestine

Rectum

Digestive Tract

Colorectal Cancer

Cancer of the colon and rectum occurs in about five percent of people over age 40. You are at increased risk if you have a family history of the disease, if you have polyps (protruding growths) in your colon, or if you have ulcerative colitis. High-fat and low-fiber diets have also been linked to colorectal cancer.

Symptoms of colorectal cancer include blood in the stool, a change in bowel movements, bleeding from the rectum, thin pencil-like stools, and lower abdominal pain. Fortunately, colorectal cancer is highly curable if recognized and treated at an early stage.

Prevention

- Eat right. Cut down on fats and increase fiber. See Chapter 20.

- Exercise on a regular basis. Physical activity keeps body wastes moving through the intestinal tract.

- Get early-detection testing:

  - Test for blood in your stool once a year. Fecal occult blood tests that can be done at home are available at drugstores. See page 347. Follow up any positive results with a physician. Professional testing is recommended every five years for those over age 50.

  - Have a digital rectal exam with every routine medical exam. This exam reaches only as far as the physician's gloved finger. It can detect only 10 percent of colorectal cancers.

  - Have a sigmoidoscopy (an exam of the rectum and colon with a flexible lighted tube) at age 50, 60, and every ten years thereafter. Sigmoidoscopy can detect 30 to 40 percent of colorectal cancers.

  - Increase the frequency of all testing if there is a family history of colon cancer, polyps, or ulcerative colitis.

When to Call a Health Professional

- If a home fecal occult blood test is positive.

- If there is bright red or red-black blood in the stool. (More than small bright red streaks from hemorrhoids or tears in the anus.)

- If there is sudden constipation or diarrhea that does not clear up with three days of home treatment. See pages 99 and 101.

- If you pass stools that are thin and pencil-like.

- If you have unexplained pain in the lower abdomen.

Constipation

Constipation occurs when bowel movements are infrequent or difficult to pass. Some people are overly concerned with frequency because they have been taught that a healthy person has a bowel movement every day. This is a misconception. Some people pass stools daily, some every three to five days; either group can be said to be "regular." If your stools are soft and pass easily, you are not constipated.

Constipation may be accompanied by cramping and pain in the rectum from the strain of trying to pass hard, dry stools. There may also be some bloating and nausea. If a stool becomes impacted, or stuck in the rectum, mucus and fluid will leak out around the stool, leading to fecal incontinence.

Older adults are somewhat more susceptible to constipation. Lack of exercise, too little fiber and fluids in the diet, laxative abuse, and some medications (antacids, antidepressants, antihistamines, diuretics, narcotics, among others) can all cause constipation.

Prevention

- Eat plenty of high-fiber foods such as fruits, vegetables, and whole grains. Three to four tablespoons of bran a day will help; add it to cereal or soups. See page 281 for more about fiber. Avoid foods that are high in fats and sugars.

- Drink 1½ to 2 quarts of water and other fluids everyday. (However, some people find milk constipating.)

- Exercise more. A walking program would be a good start. See page 262.

- Avoid overusing laxatives. They can become habit-forming. Some laxatives are also damaging to the colon. See page 335.

- Go when you feel the urge. Your bowel sends signals when there is a need to pass stools. If you ignore the signal, the urge will go away, and the stool will eventually become dry and difficult to pass.

Home Treatment

- Set aside relaxed times for bowel movements. Urges usually occur some time after meals. Establishing a daily routine, after breakfast, for example, may be helpful.

- Drink two to four extra glasses of water per day, especially in the morning.

- Add fruits, juices, and high-fiber foods to your diet.

- If necessary, use a stool softener or very mild laxative, such as milk of magnesia. Do not use mineral oil or any other laxative for more than two weeks. See page 335.

Constipation - continued

- Doctors will sometimes recommend that you take a product like Metamucil regularly. If yours does, be sure that you drink at least two quarts of water each day, remain active, and include lots of fruit and fresh vegetables in your diet.

Fecal Incontinence

The leakage of fecal matter at times other than during a bowel movement usually indicates the presence of an impacted stool in the rectum.

Stools will be less likely to become stuck if your diet contains adequate fiber, water, and bulk. See page 281 for tips on adding fiber to your diet.

When to Call a Health Professional

- If constipation persists after the above treatment is followed for one week.

- If sharp or severe pain occurs in the abdomen.

- If dark blood is seen in stools. Small amounts of bright red blood are usually caused by slight tearing as the stool is pushed through the anus. This should stop when the constipation is controlled.

More than a few streaks of bright red blood should be discussed with a health professional.

- If constipation and major changes in bowel movement patterns occur and persist without clear reason.

- If you experience fecal incontinence.

Dehydration

Dehydration is the excessive loss of water from the body. A continuous supply of water is required by all living cells in your body. Even in the resting state, your body loses water through the lungs and skin. When you stop drinking water or when you lose large amounts of fluids through diarrhea, vomiting, or sweating, body cells reabsorb fluid from the blood and other stores of water. If too much water is reabsorbed, the blood vessels collapse in vascular shock. Without medical attention, death may follow very quickly.

Because dehydration is extremely dangerous for weakened or frail people, watch closely for its signs:

- Dry mouth and excessive thirst

- A sunken eye appearance

- Little or no urine (it will be dark yellow in color)

- Dry and sticky saliva

- Inelastic skin--pinch the skin on the person's stomach. The skin will feel doughy and won't snap right back. If in doubt, compare to a well person's skin.

Home Treatment

- Treatment of mild dehydration is simple. First, stop the fluid loss. Then, restore lost fluids as soon as possible.

- If the person is nauseated or vomiting, stop all foods and fluids for two to four hours to rest the stomach.

- When vomiting is controlled, give clear liquids (water or bouillon) a sip at a time until the stomach can handle larger amounts.

- A potassium salt electrolyte solution or drink like Gatorade may be used since it will restore some of the salts lost with the fluids. Do not make it the sole source of liquids. See page 333 for a recipe you can make at home.

- Continue to check the signs of dehydration for improvement or turns for the worse.

When to Call a Health Professional

- If, after two hours of no food or liquid, the person cannot hold down even small amounts of liquid.

- If a sick, sunken eye appearance develops.

- If there has been little or no urine for 12 hours.

- If the skin is doughy.

- If a temperature of 101° or higher develops and persists more than 24 hours.

- If you cannot stop the fluid loss, the person may have to be hospitalized and given fluids intravenously.

Diarrhea

Diarrhea is an increase in the frequency of bowel movements and the discharge of watery, loose stools. The person with diarrhea may also have abdominal cramps and nausea.

Diarrhea occurs when the intestines push stools through before the water in them can be reabsorbed by the body. It is your body's way of quickly clearing out any viruses or bacteria. Most diarrhea is caused by viral or bacterial infections. Prescribed or over-the-counter medications may also upset your digestive tract enough to cause diarrhea. For some people, emotional stress and upset may bring on the condition.

Chronic or intermittent diarrhea lasting over weeks or months may be caused by one of many life-threatening conditions. Prolonged diarrhea

Diarrhea - continued

also leads to a secondary problem of malnutrition and fluid loss, since nutrients are passed before the body can absorb them. See Dehydration, page 100.

Home Treatment

- Since diarrhea may sometimes speed recovery of the underlying problem, avoid anti-diarrheal drugs for the first six hours. After that, use them only if cramping or discomfort continues. See the discussion on anti-diarrheal preparations on page 332.

- Put your stomach at rest. Drink only clear liquids for the first 24 hours.

- Begin eating mild foods, such as rice, bananas, and applesauce the next day. Spicy foods, fruit, alcohol, and coffee should be avoided until 48 hours after all symptoms have disappeared. Avoid dairy products for three days.

When to Call a Health Professional

- If stools are bloody or black. However, Pepto-Bismol or other medications containing bismuth will cause stools to look tarry.

- If diarrhea lasts for three days or more.

- If abdominal pain or severe discomfort accompanies diarrhea and is not immediately relieved by the passage of stools or gas.

- If diarrhea is accompanied by fever of 101° or higher, chills, vomiting, or fainting.

- If signs of dehydration appear. See page 100.

Diverticulosis/ Diverticulitis

Many older people have diverticulosis (diver-tick-u-low-sis), a condition in which small sacs form on the wall of the colon. These pouches generally cause no symptoms, although there may be occasional pain

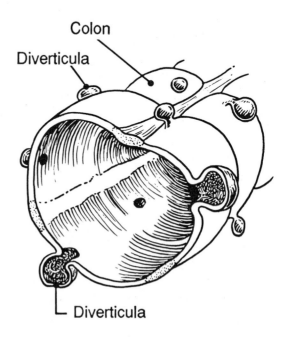

Colon

Diverticula

Diverticula

Diverticulosis

in the lower left side of the abdomen. Diverticulosis is not a serious problem.

If the pouches and surrounding area become inflamed, the condition is renamed diverticulitis. Symptoms include crampy pain, usually in the lower left abdomen, constipation, and fever. A doctor will need to be consulted.

Prevention

- Keep your colon in good health by eating the right foods and drinking 1½ to 2 quarts of water each day. Eat more fruits, vegetables, and whole-grain breads. Add three to four tablespoons of wheat bran to your daily diet. See page 281 for more on fiber. When adding more fiber, add more liquid--at least two quarts every day.

- Avoid constipation and don't strain during bowel movements.

- Avoid laxatives.

- Avoid drugs that slow down bowel action, such as painkillers and antidepressants.

When to Call a Health Professional

- If there is severe and increasing abdominal pain, especially when associated with fever.

- If stools are red or red-black in color.

Food Poisoning/ Stomach Flu

Food poisoning and stomach flu are different ailments with different causes. However, most people confuse the two because the symptoms are so similar. Most people who get food poisoning attribute their symptoms of nausea, vomiting, diarrhea, and severe pain to a sudden case of stomach flu, and vice versa. The home treatment is the same for both problems.

Stomach flu is usually caused by a viral infection in the digestive system, hence the medical name, viral gastroenteritis.

Bacterial or viral, the infection brings on disagreeable symptoms-- stomach pain, diarrhea, nausea, and vomiting--to discourage you from eating until the problem clears up.

Food poisoning is caused by a bacterial infection. When certain foods, particularly meats and dairy products, are left at temperatures between 40° and 140°, the bacteria in them thrive and grow rapidly. The bacteria produce a poison or toxin that causes an acute inflammation of the intestines. The violence of the illness varies with the amount of toxin in the body and with individual susceptibility.

To determine if the illness is food poisoning, ask:

Food Poisoning - continued

- Has the person shared a meal with anyone with similar symptoms?

- Has the person consumed an unusual amount or type of food or drink?

- Has the person eaten any unrefrigerated meat recently?

Most food poisoning occurs during the summer when picnickers eat unrefrigerated meats, or on special occasions when cold cuts, turkey, dressing, sauces, and other foods are not kept under 40° or above 140°. Other problems arise if foods are not prepared properly during home canning. If any bacteria survive the canning process,they may grow and produce toxin in the can or jar.

The symptoms of food poisoning do not begin immediately; 6 to 48 hours may pass before the onset of the symptoms. Illness may last from 12 hours to two days for common food poisoning.

Botulism, although rare, is fatal in 65 percent of cases. It is generally caused by improper home canning methods for low-acid foods like beans and corn. Symptoms include blurred vision, inability to swallow, and progressive difficulty in breathing.

Prevention

- To prevent stomach flu, you must avoid contact with the virus--not always an easy thing to do.

- To prevent food poisoning:

  o Follow the 2-40-140 Rule. Don't eat meats, dressing, or sauces that have been kept between 40° and 140° for more than two hours.

  o Be especially careful with large cooked meats like your holiday turkey, which require a long time to cool. Some parts of the meat may stay over 40° long enough to produce bacteria.

  o Use a thermometer to check your refrigerator. It should be between 34° and 40°.

  o Defrost meats in the refrigerator or the microwave, not on the kitchen counter.

  o Reheat meats to over 140° for ten minutes to destroy bacteria. Even then, the toxin may not be destroyed.

  o Put party foods on ice to keep them cool.

  o Discard any cans or jars with bulging lids or leaks.

- Wash your hands, cutting boards, and counter tops frequently. Acrylic cutting boards are safer than wood.

- Cover meats and poultry during microwave cooking to heat the surface of the meat.

- Follow home canning and freezing instructions to the letter. Call your County Agricultural Extension office for advice.

- When you eat out, avoid rare and uncooked meats. Eat salad bar and deli items immediately.

Home Treatment

For both stomach flu and food poisoning:

- Do not eat or drink until vomiting has stopped. Ice chips and small sips of water are okay.

- Drink clear non-carbonated liquids only for 24 hours. Start with a few sips at a time.

- Gradually progress to easily digestible foods such as applesauce and Jell-O.

- Avoid spicy foods, dairy products, alcohol, and coffee for 48 hours after all symptoms have gone.

- If you suspect food poisoning, check with others who may have eaten the same food. If possible, save a sample of the suspected food for analysis in case symptoms do not improve.

When to Call a Health Professional

- If you cannot control vomiting after 12 hours of ice chips only.

- If there is fever of 101° or higher.

- If vomiting or diarrhea is severe.

- If diarrhea continues after 48 hours of a liquids-only diet or if stools are bloody or black.

- If the pain is severe, increases, or continues for over four hours.

- If mild but continuous pain lasts over 12 hours.

- If you suspect food poisoning from a canned product or have any of the symptoms of botulism poisoning (blurred vision, difficulty in swallowing or breathing). Take suspect food with you if you still have it.

Gallbladder Disease

The gallbladder is a small sac attached to the underside of the liver. It stores bile produced by the liver to help your body digest fats. If the bile becomes too concentrated, gallstones can develop. The gallstones may lie quietly in the gallbladder causing no problems. However, a stone may

Gallbladder Disease - continued

cause the gallbladder to become inflamed. The pain from a gallstone attack is centered under the right rib cage. Fever and vomiting may also be present.

Gallstones may also cause problems by moving out of the gallbladder and getting stuck in the bile duct. The backup of bile in the system will cause the skin and whites of the eyes to take on a yellow tint (jaundice). The urine may turn dark brown. There will also be severe pain, fever, and vomiting.

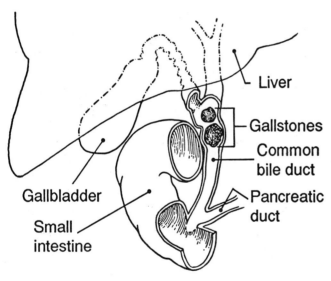

Gallbladder

Women are far more likely than men to develop gallbladder disease; between 20 percent and 25 percent of all women over age 55 have gallstones. Other risk factors include obesity, a diet high in fat and sugar, rapid weight loss, lack of exercise, diabetes, hypertension, and estrogen replacement therapy. For unknown reasons, Native American women are particularly high-risk candidates for gallstones.

The best way to avoid the pain and complications of gallbladder disease is to reduce your risk.

Prevention

- Eat wholesome foods. Follow a diet high in fiber and low in fats, sugars, and cholesterol. Chapter 20 contains helpful hints.

- Maintain ideal weight.

- Avoid crash diets. Rapid weight loss greatly increases the risk of gallstones.

- Exercise. It's never too late and the benefits are worth the effort. See Chapter 19.

- Quit smoking. See page 76.

- Talk with your doctor about the pros and cons of estrogen replacement therapy if you are considering such a course. See page 211.

Home Treatment

If you develop gallstones, follow the prevention guidelines above. They will help keep the problem from getting worse.

When to Call a Health Professional

- The first time you experience pain from gallstones--pain and tenderness in the upper right portion of your abdomen.

- If skin takes on a yellowish tint.

- If urine is dark-brown.

- If you are obese and plan a rapid weight-loss program. Medications can help prevent gallstone formation.

Heartburn/ Indigestion

Heartburn is caused by stomach acids backing up into the lower esophagus, the tube that leads from the mouth to the stomach. The acids produce a burning sensation and discomfort between the ribs just below the breastbone. Heartburn can occur after overeating or sometimes in reaction to medications.

Don't be concerned if you experience heartburn now and then; nearly everyone does. However, repeated episodes of heartburn can injure the esophageal lining.

Prevention

- Don't overeat. Avoid late-night meals.

- Avoid tight-fitting clothes, such as belts and girdles.

- Avoid constipation, since it can increase pressure on the stomach. See page 99.

- Try acetaminophen (Tylenol) instead of aspirin and ibuprofen, which may cause heartburn.

- Prevent future attacks by taking note of what foods or beverages bring on distress. If certain foods seem to cause trouble, avoid them. Alcohol, caffeine, chocolate, peppermint, and citrus fruits and juices are common culprits. If you can draw a connection, you may be able to prevent future attacks by avoiding the substance.

- Stop smoking. Nicotine weakens the opening at the top of the stomach and is directly related to heartburn.

Home Treatment

- Discontinue alcohol, nicotine, chocolate, caffeine, and fatty foods since all of them weaken the valve that keeps stomach acid out of the esophagus.

- Avoid acidic foods such as citrus fruits, tomatoes, and vinegar.

- Don't lie down too soon after eating. Try to stay upright for at least two to three hours after each meal.

- Raise the head of your bed four to six inches using wooden blocks or thick telephone books.

Heartburn - continued

- Take an antacid, such as Maalox, Mylanta, or Gelusil, but use it wisely. See page 331.

When to Call a Health Professional

- If the problem lasts for more than three days. Call sooner if symptoms are not relieved at all by antacids. See Ulcers, page 111.

- If you suspect that a prescribed medication is causing the heartburn. Antihistamines, Valium, and ibuprofen sometimes cause heartburn.

- If shortness of breath or other symptoms suggest heart problems. See Chest Pain, page 64.

Hemorrhoids/ Rectal Itching

Hemorrhoids and piles are two terms used to describe inflammation and swelling of the veins around the anus. Hemorrhoids may be located either inside or outside the anus. Straining to pass hard, compacted stools sometimes irritates these veins. The symptoms of hemorrhoids are rectal itching, tenderness or pain, and sometimes bleeding. They generally last several days.

Rectal itching may also be caused by other conditions. Skin may become irritated by any fecal seepage that comes with diarrhea or loss of bowel control. If the anus is not kept clean, itching may result. Too much rubbing with dry toilet paper may injure the skin, too.

Prevention

- Keep your stools soft. Include plenty of water, fresh fruits and vegetables, whole grains, and beans in your diet.

- Avoid sitting too much. This restricts blood flow around your anus.

- Try not to strain during bowel movements. Take your time and never hold your breath.

Home Treatment

- Keep the area clean. Warm baths are soothing and cleansing, especially after a bowel movement. Try premoistened tissues (baby wipes) instead of toilet paper.

- Wear cotton underwear and loose clothing.

- Apply zinc oxide (paste or powder) or Vaseline to the painful area after drying. This protects against further irritation and eases the passage of stools.

- Relieve itching by using cold compresses on the anus four times a day, ten minutes at a time.

- The following over-the-counter preparations may help: Tucks, Balneol, or stool softeners. Avoid anal ointments with a local anesthetic compound. These will have the suffix "caine" in the name or ingredients.

- Take aspirin or use medicated suppositories to relieve pain.

When to Call a Health Professional

- If pain is severe or lasts longer than one week.

- If bleeding continues or is heavy, or if the blood is dark in color.

Irritable Bowel Syndrome

Irritable bowel syndrome is a common digestive complaint. It is not linked to any serious illness; the intestinal tract is just not working properly. Symptoms include abdominal pain, gas, bloating, diarrhea, or constipation.

Stress seems to trigger episodes of irritable bowel syndrome. Diet is also involved. Sensitivities to milk, wheat, eggs, potatoes, and certain other foods are found among 15 percent of people who suffer from this ailment.

Prevention

- Manage your stress. See Chapter 21.

- Relieve physical tension through exercise. See Chapter 19.

Controlling Intestinal Gas

Passing intestinal gas, even as much as twenty times per day, is perfectly normal. However, if you want to reduce flatulence, there are some things you can do.

- Don't give up on beans; they are too good for you. Soak dry beans overnight, but use fresh water for cooking. Cook beans thoroughly.

- If dairy products give you gas, switch to cultured milk products (yogurt and buttermilk) or add a lactase supplement (Lact-Aid) to your milk to help your digestion.

- Read labels for two sweeteners, fructose and sorbitol. They may cause an increase in flatulence.

- Don't bolt your food. Large lumps of food are harder to digest.

- Avoid constipation by eating a high-fiber diet and drinking plenty of water.

Irritable Bowel - continued

- Watch your diet. Tips for dietary control of irritable bowel syndrome include:

  ○ Cut back on all fats in your diet. See page 285.

  ○ Eat more fiber. See page 281.

  ○ Plan meals that are low in fat and high in carbohydrates. Include vegetables, fruits, whole-grain breads and cereals, pasta, and rice.

Home Treatment

- Follow the prevention guidelines above.

- If cramps and diarrhea occur, eating smaller meals throughout the day may ease the strain on your colon.

- If symptoms appear after eating certain foods, try eliminating those foods from your diet.

When to Call a Health Professional

- If pain and discomfort do not respond to home treatment.

- If blood appears in the stool.

Nausea and Vomiting

Nausea is a very unpleasant sensation in the pit of the stomach. A person with nausea may feel weak and sweaty. Lots of saliva may be produced. Intense nausea often leads to vomiting.

Vomiting forces stomach contents up the esophagus and out the mouth. Most vomiting is caused by viral infections. Home treatment will help ease the discomfort.

In older adults, vomiting is often a sign of a medication reaction. Nausea and vomiting can also be symptoms of other serious illnesses. Be concerned if nausea and vomiting persist; older adults can become dehydrated very quickly with fluid loss from vomiting. See Dehydration, page 100.

Home Treatment

- Take nothing by mouth for four hours after the onset of vomiting. Ice chips and small sips of water may be all right.

- Drink only clear non-carbonated liquids such as water or broth for 24 hours. Start with a few sips at a time and gradually increase.

- Rest in bed until aches subside.

- Eat only soups, mild foods, and liquids on the second day and until all symptoms are gone for 48 hours.

When to Call a Health Professional

- If you suspect that medication is causing the problem. Know which of your medications can cause nausea or vomiting.

- If nausea and vomiting last for more than two days.

- If vomiting is severe or violent. (It shoots out in large quantities.)

- If there is blood in the vomit; it may look like red or black coffee grounds.

- If nausea or vomiting is preventing you from taking medications you need for chronic conditions, such as high blood pressure.

- If signs of dehydration appear. See page 100.

- If nausea or vomiting occurs after a head injury.

Ulcers

An ulcer is a sore or lesion in the inside lining of the gastrointestinal tract. Ulcers appear when there is too much stomach acid or when the mucous lining protecting the digestive tract is abnormal. There is also evidence that bacteria that damage

the stomach lining may lead to chronic ulcers.

Older adults who take anti-inflammatory drugs (aspirin, ibuprofen, naproxen) for arthritis are at increased risk for ulcers.

There are two kinds of ulcers: gastric, which appear in the stomach, and duodenal, which form in the duodenum (the first part of the small intestine). It is possible to have both kinds of ulcers at the same time.

Symptoms of a duodenal ulcer may include a burning or sharp pain in the region just above the navel. The burning pain is usually strongest when the stomach is empty. People with these ulcers are sometimes awakened by pain in the middle of the night. Eating a slice of plain bread will

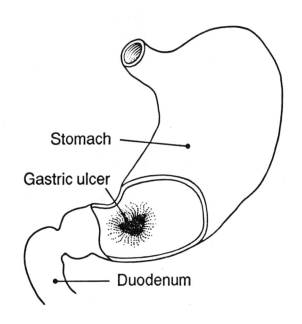

Stomach

Gastric ulcer

Duodenum

Ulcer

Ulcers - continued

usually relieve the pain by neutralizing the acid for a while. (Avoid milk. Some studies show that milk interferes with the healing of an ulcer.)

The dull aching pain of gastric ulcers is located above the navel. Nausea and vomiting may also be present. Eating generally does not bring relief.

If undetected or left untreated, ulcers can lead to peritonitis, an inflammation of the lining of the abdominal cavity.

Prevention

- Slow down. Stress contributes to ulcers. For help managing your stress levels, see Chapter 21.

- Quit smoking. Tobacco smoke constricts the small vessels lining the stomach, making the stomach wall more vulnerable to sores.

- Discuss your use of aspirin and anti-inflammatory drugs with your doctor or pharmacist. Some studies have linked these and other medications with an increased risk of ulcers.

Home Treatment

- When you first suspect you have an ulcer, try to heal it quickly. Take a few days to relax and improve your diet. You may avoid an expensive hospitalization later.

- Change your diet. Eliminate alcohol and reduce caffeine to absolute minimums. Eat more often (four to six light meals a day).

- Cut out foods that seem to make symptoms worse.

- Stop smoking.

- Avoid aspirin and ibuprofen (Advil).

- Antacids are usually necessary to neutralize your gastric acids long enough for your ulcer to heal. You need frequent and large amounts of antacids to do the job. Talk with your health professional about how much to take. Nonabsorbable antacids like Maalox, Mylanta, or Gelusil are often best. Most antacids have a high salt content and should be used with caution by persons on low-sodium diets or people with high blood pressure. People with diabetes should be aware that some antacids contain glucose. See page 331.

When to Call a Health Professional

- To diagnose and evaluate a suspected ulcer. An examination, history, and test can often determine the presence, location, and severity of an ulcer.

- To determine appropriate antacid dosage.

- If you are suddenly weak or dizzy.

- If vomiting accompanies pain.

- If vomit contains blood or material that looks like coffee grounds.

- If black, tarry blood appears in the stool.

- If severe pain is not relieved by your treatment program.

Urinary Incontinence

If you suffer from urinary incontinence (loss of bladder control), you are not alone. At least 10 to 20 percent of all older adults living in the community are coping with this problem.

Many cases of incontinence can be controlled, if not cured outright. Temporary incontinence can be caused by water pills (diuretics) and many other common medications. Constipation, urinary infections, stones in the urinary tract, or extended bed rest are other causes. If the underlying problem is corrected, the incontinence can be cured.

There are five types of persistent or chronic loss of bladder control:

Stress incontinence refers to small amounts of urine leaking out during exercise, coughing, laughing, sneezing, or other movements that squeeze the bladder. It is most often seen in women, although men may experience it after prostate surgery.

This kind of incontinence is often helped by Kegel exercises. See page 114.

Urge incontinence happens when the need to urinate comes on so quickly there is not enough time to get to the toilet. Stroke, Parkinson's disease, kidney or bladder stones, and bladder infection are some of the causes of urge incontinence.

Overflow incontinence occurs when the bladder cannot empty itself completely. Diabetes or an enlarged prostate may be the underlying cause.

Reflex incontinence is spontaneous urination without the feeling of needing to go. Spinal cord injury, diabetes, multiple sclerosis, and other ailments cause this lack of bladder control.

Functional incontinence may occur in people who have bladder control but have difficulty getting to the bathroom quickly enough because of physical limitations.

Home Treatment

- Don't let incontinence embarrass you. It is not a sign of approaching senility. Take charge and work with your doctor to treat any underlying conditions that may be causing the problem.

- Don't let incontinence keep you from doing the things you like to do. Absorbent pads or briefs, such

Incontinence - continued

as Attends and Depend, are available in pharmacies and supermarkets. No one will know you are wearing one.

- Avoid coffee, tea, and other drinks that contain caffeine, which overstimulates the bladder. Do not cut down on overall fluids; you need these to keep the rest of your body healthy.

- Practice "double-voiding." Empty your bladder as much as possible, relax for a minute, and then try to empty your bladder again.

- Urinate on a schedule, perhaps every three to four hours during the day, whether the urge is there or not. This may help you to restore control.

- Wear clothing that can be easily removed, such as pants with elastic waistbands. If you have difficulty with buttons and zippers, consider replacing them with velcro closures.

- Keep skin in the genital area dry to prevent rashes. Vaseline or Desitin ointment will help.

- Pay special attention to any medications you are taking, including over-the-counter drugs, since some affect bladder control.

- Incontinence is sometimes caused by a urinary tract infection. If you feel pain or burning when you urinate, see the home treatment for urinary tract infection on page 116.

- For stress incontinence, practice Kegel exercises daily. See below.

Kegel Exercises

Kegel exercises can help cure or improve stress incontinence. They strengthen the muscles that control the flow of urine.

- Locate the muscles by repeatedly stopping your urine in mid-stream and starting again. The muscles that you feel squeezing around your urethra and anus are the ones to focus on.

- Practice squeezing these muscles while you are not urinating. If your stomach or buttocks move, you are not using the right muscles.

- Hold the squeeze for three seconds--then relax for three seconds.

- Repeat the exercise 10 to 15 times per session.

- Do at least three Kegel exercise sessions per day.

Kegel exercises are simple and effective. You can do them anywhere and anytime. No one will know you are doing them except you.

- Ease functional incontinence by placing a portable commode where it can be reached easily, such as by your bed.

For more information on urinary incontinence, see Resources O1-2 on page 350 or contact Help for Incontinent People, P.O. Box 544, Union, SC 29379, (803)579-7900.

When to Call a Health Professional

- If you experience more than one episode of urinary incontinence, even in small amounts.

- If you feel that you cannot completely empty your bladder.

An infection of the urethra is known as urethritis. Cystitis is a bladder infection and nephritis is the term for kidney infection. See the warning signs of a kidney infection on page 116.

Symptoms of urethritis and cystitis are urgent and frequent urination, a burning sensation during voiding, itching, or pain in the urethra. The urine may be cloudy or reddish in color. Chills and fever may also be present if the infection is severe.

Men with similar symptoms may be experiencing an infection of the prostate gland. See page 221.

Urinary Tract Infections

The urinary tract is composed of the kidneys, ureters, bladder, and urethra. Urine is formed by the kidneys as they filter waste products from the blood. The urine is carried from the kidneys to the bladder through the ureters. The bladder holds the urine until it is expelled through the urethra. The system may become irritated and inflamed by viruses, bacteria, or even too much caffeine.

The inflammation of any part of this system by bacteria is known as a urinary tract infection.

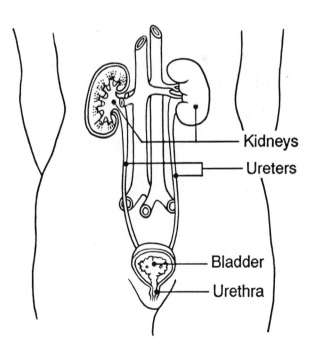

Urinary Tract

Urinary Tract Infections - cont'd

Men who have enlarged prostates, women who have had multiple pregnancies, and people with kidney stones or diabetes may be at more risk for repeated infections.

Because the organs of the urinary tract are connected, infection can easily spread from one organ to the next. If left untreated, some infections may go on to the kidneys and cause permanent kidney damage. Because of this danger, pain upon urination should always be treated promptly.

Prevention

- Drink more fluids--water is good.

- Urinate frequently.

- Women should wipe from front to back after going to the toilet. This will reduce the spread of bacteria from the rectum to the urethra.

- Avoid frequent douching and do not use vaginal deodorants or perfumed feminine hygiene products.

- Women susceptible to urinary infections should urinate before and after intercourse. Drinking extra water after intercourse may also help prevent infection.

- Wear cotton underwear, cotton-lined pantyhose, and loose clothing.

Home Treatment

- Drink as much water or fruit juice (think in terms of gallons) as you can in the first 24 hours after symptoms appear. This will help clear out the infection.

- Avoid alcohol, coffee, and spicy foods.

- Get extra rest.

- If you suffer from frequent urinary tract infections, use a home test to detect *E. coli* bacteria in the urine. You can buy nitrate dip strips and urine dip cultures at a pharmacy. If bacteria are found, antibiotics will need to be prescribed.

When to Call a Health Professional

- If there is no improvement after 24 hours of home treatment.

Warning Signs of Kidney Problems

Call a health professional if these symptoms appear:

- Bloody or tea-colored urine

- Lower back pain just below the rib cage

- Swelling in the ankles (edema)

- Puffiness around the eyes

- Increased frequency of urination

- High blood pressure

- If pain on urination is accompanied by any of the following symptoms:

  - Chills and/or fever of 101° or higher

  - Inability to urinate when you feel the urge

  - Pain or tenderness in the thighs

  - Low back pain

  - Bloody or tea-colored urine (Note: Beets and certain medications can cause urine to be red the next day.)

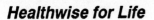

"Yes, I am an old enemy of the human race, but I am not that unbeatable once my name is said," spoke the Pale Stranger.
From a Native American story about diabetes by John McLeod

7

Diabetes and Thyroid Problems

Your endocrine system serves as a control system for your body. The glands that make up the endocrine system include the pituitary, the thyroid and parathyroid, the pancreas, the adrenal glands, the ovaries, and the testes. Each of these glands secretes special hormones, or chemical messengers, that help your body's organs do their jobs.

This chapter focuses on two common endocrine disorders: diabetes and thyroid problems. These problems are very responsive to prevention and self-help. By following good health practices and early detection measures, you can help your endocrine system function at its best.

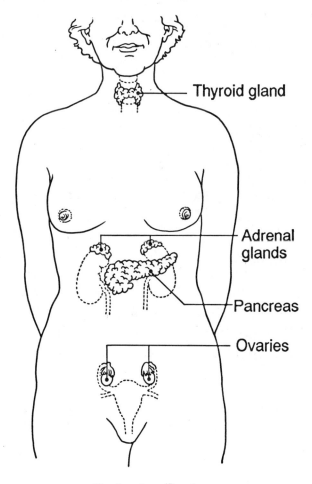

Thyroid gland

Adrenal glands

Pancreas

Ovaries

Endocrine System

Diabetes

When you pull up to the gas pump you have your choice of fuels: regular, unleaded, super, or diesel. Your body, on the other hand, uses only one fuel to run each and every cell. This fuel is glucose. The starches and sugars in the food you eat are converted to glucose before your body uses it.

Insulin is a hormone released by the pancreas to control the amount of glucose in the blood. Without insulin, the body cannot use or store glucose.

Insulin is released when blood glucose levels are high (usually after a meal). The insulin allows some glucose into cells where it is converted into energy. It helps other glucose to be stored in fat and muscle cells for later use. Excess glucose is also stored in the liver. In a healthy body, insulin keeps the amount of glucose in the blood under tight control.

Diabetes results from a breakdown in this system, which leads to a higher than normal amount of glucose in the blood. There are two types of diabetes; each is quite different.

Type I, or insulin-dependent diabetes mellitus (IDDM), occurs when the pancreas fails to make enough insulin to keep blood glucose levels in balance. Type I diabetes generally occurs in childhood or adolescence. However, it can develop at any age. People with this kind of diabetes must inject insulin every day.

Type II, or noninsulin-dependent diabetes mellitus (NIDDM), occurs when body cells become somewhat resistant to insulin. This reduces the amount of glucose that can be used by the cells at any one time. Type II diabetes is the most common form among older adults (particularly those who are overweight).

Many people with type II diabetes are able to control their blood sugar through weight control, regular exercise, and a sensible diet. Others may need insulin injections or medications taken by mouth to lower blood sugar (oral hypoglycemic agents).

Anyone with any two of the following risk factors has an increased chance of developing type II diabetes:

- Age 40 or over

- Overweight

- Family history of diabetes

- African-American, Hispanic, or Native American

Symptoms of Diabetes

Most of the symptoms of diabetes are vague and, by themselves, seldom lead to a physician visit. These symptoms include:

- Increased thirst

- Frequent urination

- Increased appetite

- Unexplained weight loss

- Fatigue

- Skin infections

- Slow-healing wounds

- Recurrent episodes of vaginitis

- Difficulty with erections

- Blurred vision

- Tingling or numbness in hands or feet

Only a blood glucose test done by a health professional can accurately diagnose diabetes. Blood glucose tests are inexpensive and very low-risk. Ask your doctor if you should eat or fast before the test.

Complications of Diabetes

Diabetes has two types of long-term effects: damage to blood vessels and damage to nerves. Because of these complications, the person with diabetes is at higher risk for:

- Atherosclerosis, hypertension, and heart disease

- Stroke

- Visual problems and blindness (See Diabetic Retinopathy on page 156.)

- Kidney failure

- Loss of a limb

Early diagnosis and control of diabetes is important to prevent serious complications. If you are at increased risk for diabetes, have a blood glucose test once each year.

Prevention

At this time there is no known way of effectively preventing type I diabetes. In most cases the risk of type II diabetes can be reduced by regular, daily exercise (see Chapter 19) and weight control (see Chapter 20).

Home Treatment

There are nine key points to follow for home treatment of both type I and type II diabetes.

1. Get in control.

"You have diabetes." These words can be discouraging. They can make you feel shock, anger, fear, sadness, and guilt--all at the same time. You may fear that diabetes means the start of a gradual slide into poor health. You may feel overwhelmed.

It doesn't help to hear all of the things that you must do:

- Lose weight

- Start exercising

- Stop smoking

- Reduce stress

- Control your diet

- Take your medication

Diabetes - continued

If it all feels hopeless, take heart. People with diabetes do not have to become "sick." You can win control over diabetes by making one small change at a time.

Step 1: Start with a positive vision of yourself. Read about mental wellness on page 305. If you can raise your expectations about becoming more healthy, it will be much easier to accomplish.

Step 2: Pick out one behavior from the list of "must-dos" above. Choose the one that you think you can improve most easily and start there. Develop a step-by-step plan for success.

That's it; there is no Step 3. Just keep repeating Step 2 until you are as healthy as you want to be.

2. Take care of your feet.

Proper foot care is important for people with diabetes. The disease impairs nerve function and limits blood flow to the feet. Small cuts, sores, and even ingrown toenails can quickly become seriously infected.

- Wash feet daily with warm water and mild soap. Dry well.

- Avoid strong chemicals such as epsom salts, iodine, and corn removers.

- Inspect the feet while drying. Pay special attention to any signs of cuts, cracking, or peeling between the toes or on the bottom of the foot.

- Use lanolin or other moisturizers to keep the skin soft.

- Cut and file toenails straight across.

- Break in new shoes slowly to avoid blisters.

- Don't walk barefoot, even indoors. It's too easy to bruise or cut your feet.

- Stop smoking. Smoking reduces blood flow even more.

- Call your doctor if you have any of the following:

  - Ingrown toenail

  - Athlete's foot

  - New corn or callus

  - A bunion that is irritated by chafing from shoes

  - A cut, sore, or discoloration that shows no sign of healing. Prescription antibiotics may be needed to prevent serious infection.

3. Get regular eye exams.

Changes in the eye that are caused by diabetes often have no symptoms until they are quite advanced. Early treatment of diabetic retinopathy may slow its progress and save your sight. See page 156.

4. Eat a healthful diet.

People with diabetes need a healthful diet for two reasons. First, a proper diet helps keep your blood sugar levels in control. Second, a good diet helps with weight control, and being close to your ideal weight reduces your risk of type II diabetes.

See Chapter 20 for basic guidelines for healthy food choices. In general, the person with diabetes needs to:

- Eat less fat.

- Eat more high-fiber foods, such as whole-grain breads, vegetables, and fruit.

- Use less salt.

- Avoid simple sugars, such as table sugar, honey, candy, and sugary drinks. These are absorbed into the bloodstream too rapidly.

- Limit alcohol to no more than one drink per day

- Spread calories out over four to six meals, for example, three small meals with three snacks. Try to avoid eating a lot of food at one meal, which could overload the blood with glucose.

- Switching to a healthful diet may reduce your need for anti-diabetic medications. Ask your doctor.

5. Get active.

Regular aerobic exercise will help you regulate your blood sugar, reduce your risk of heart disease, and control your weight--all essential ingredients to good diabetes management. However, people with diabetes also need to be aware of how exercise affects their blood glucose levels.

Before beginning an exercise program, work with your doctor to identify any complications, such as poor circulation or nerve damage, that might pose a serious risk. Your physician can help you develop an exercise program suited to your needs. It helps to measure your blood sugar before and after exercise for several days.

Plan to check back with your doctor after any increase in regular exercise. The more you exercise, the less medication you may need.

6. Track your diabetes for 30 days.

The key to managing diabetes is careful monitoring of your blood glucose levels. In 30 days, you can learn how your diet and activities affect your blood sugar.

Ask your doctor to recommend a home blood sugar test. Both urine dip strips and finger prick tests are available for home use. Your doctor will help you determine when, how often, and what kind of test is best for you. Keep careful records of the results of each test.

Use a journal to record these items every day for 30 days:

- The time and content of each meal

Diabetes - continued

- The kind and amount of exercise you get

- How tired or energetic you feel

- Your blood sugar level at least once a day at different times each day

This may seem inconvenient in the short term, but it will provide you with a lifelong tool for controlling your diabetes. Once you understand how your body reacts to different foods and exercise, you can correct glucose imbalances before they get out of control. After the 30-day trial, use the journal for occasional spot checks.

7. Manage your medications.

Type II diabetes is generally managed without medications. However, your doctor may prescribe an anti-diabetic drug for you if diet alone is not working. This medication must be taken as prescribed. Not enough medication will make your blood sugar higher than normal; too much will make it lower than normal. Consistency is important. As you improve your diet and exercise, your need for medication may diminish. Check with your physician.

8. Join a support group.

Diabetes support groups can add a lot to your home treatment. These groups are made up of people with diabetes and supportive health professionals. They are usually offered without cost and are excellent sources of the information needed for successful diabetes management. A local hospital should have information. Also ask about diabetes education programs available in your community.

9. Be a partner with your doctor.

You and your doctor need to work as a team. Your job is to make improvements in exercise and diet, practice good foot care, do regular glucose testing at home, keep a journal, and report all changes to your doctor.

Your doctor's job is to help you understand your illness, adjust your medications as your needs change, and treat complications before they become serious. Together, you and your doctor can control your diabetes.

For more information about diabetes management, see Resource L1 on page 350.

The National Diabetes Information Clearinghouse (Box NDIC, 9000 Rockville Pike, Bethesda, MD 20892), is a good resource for more information on diabetes management.

When to Call a Health Professional

- For a blood glucose test, if you suspect diabetes but are undiagnosed. See symptoms on page 120.

Diabetic Emergencies*

	Hypoglycemia (Low blood sugar)	Hyperglycemia (High blood sugar)
Who	Those who take insulin or an oral anti-diabetic medication	Any person with diabetes
Onset	Rapidly, over minutes or hours	Gradually, over days
Blood test	Under 70mg/% sugar	Over 300mg/% sugar
Urine test	No sugar	High sugar
Symptoms	Fatigue, weakness, nausea Hunger Sweating Double or blurred vision Pounding heart Confusion, irritability, appearance of drunkenness Loss of consciousness (insulin shock)	Frequent urination Intense thirst Dry skin Dim vision Rapid breathing Fruity-smelling breath Loss of consciousness (diabetic coma/ketoacidosis)
What to do?	Eat or drink something containing sugar. If symptoms recur, go to emergency room.	Call doctor or go directly to emergency room.

*If you are unsure about the cause of the diabetic emergency in a person who uses insulin, always give the person something containing sugar, such as candy, sugar under the tongue, orange juice, or a soft drink with sugar. Do not give an unconscious person food or drink.

Diabetes - continued

- If there are signs of changes in your normal blood sugar levels:

  o Unexplained changes in home glucose tests

  o Increased thirst, urination, or appetite

  o Unexplained weight loss

  o Continuing low blood sugar symptoms (See page 125.)

  o A change in mental functioning (confusion, drowsiness, agitation)

- For any infection:

  o Skin infections

  o Genital infections

  o Urinary tract infections

  o Ear infections

- **For diabetic emergencies (diabetic coma and insulin shock), get immediate medical attention. See page 125.**

Thyroid Problems

The thyroid is located in the front of the neck, just below the Adam's apple. This gland functions as a kind of "throttle" for the body. As the thyroid gland releases more hormone, the body runs faster. As the hormone decreases, the body slows down.

Thyroid problems are common among older people, but often go undetected. The symptoms may develop so slowly that you do not notice them, or you may dismiss them as part of "normal aging."

The thyroid can cause problems in two ways: by producing too much hormone, or by producing too little. Symptoms of too much thyroid hormone, or a hyperthyroid gland, include:

- Weight loss despite increased appetite

- Intolerance of heat

- Alternating periods of constipation and diarrhea

- Itchy, irritated, and puffy eyes

- Rapid pulse and/or palpitations

- Unexplained shortness of breath, or difficulty breathing while lying down

- Night sweats

- Progressive muscle weakness, especially in the large muscles of the legs

- Anxiety, irritability, depression, forgetfulness

- Swelling of the thyroid gland itself, often called "goiter"

These symptoms are often confused with those of other diseases. A hyperthyroid is easily detected with a simple blood test. When medical treatment is complete, thyroid function usually returns to normal.

Symptoms that the thyroid is producing too little hormone (hypothyroid) include:

- Intolerance of cold

- Constipation

- Slowed heartbeat and reflexes

- Forgetfulness, depression, lethargy, or confusion

- Chronic fatigue

- Swelling of the face, tongue, and vocal chords. Sometimes the voice grows progressively deeper.

- An underactive thyroid can also swell and form a goiter.

Treatment of a hypothyroid gland is quite simple. Your doctor can prescribe a medication that acts like real thyroid hormone in your body. In most cases, this medication will be taken for life.

Prevention

- A thyroid function test can detect changes in the amount of thyroid hormone in your body, even before you have noticed symptoms. Annual tests are recommended for:

  - People with a family history of thyroid problems

  - Women over age 65

  - Anyone with a history of radiation treatment

- One test every five years is recommended for men over 65.

Home Treatment

- If you have a prescription for daily thyroid medications, take them every day.

When to Call a Health Professional

- If any of the symptoms listed above cause you to suspect that you have a thyroid function problem.

- If a person with a hyperthyroid develops the following symptoms:

  - Fever

  - Extreme weakness

  - Rapid or irregular heart rate and pulse

  - Profuse sweating

  - Restlessness, agitation, or delirium

  - Shock, unconsciousness, or coma

Thyroid Problems - continued

- If the following symptoms
  develop, especially in a person
  with diagnosed hypothyroid:

  - Extreme intolerance of cold

  - Lethargy and fatigue that
    progresses to unconsciousness

I'm very brave generally, only today I
happen to have a headache.
Tweedledum in "Alice in Wonderland"

8

Headaches

Headache is one of the most common health complaints. It can be caused by a number of things: tension, exposure to chemicals, infection, injury, hunger, or changes in the flow of blood in the vessels of the head.

Most headaches that occur without other symptoms will respond well to self-care. The information in this chapter will help you treat common headaches at home, as well as provide tips on how you may be able to prevent them from recurring.

Sometimes, a headache can be a symptom of a serious health problem that requires the attention of a health professional. See "Headache Emergencies" on this page if you have an unusual or very severe headache.

Headache Emergencies

Call your physician now if you experience:

- A severe and sudden "thunderclap" headache

- Severe and stabbing head pain

- A blow to the head that results in severe pain, enlarged pupils, lethargy, confusion, or vomiting

- Severe head pain in combination with a stiff neck, fever, or vomiting

- Head pain combined with any vision disturbances

- Head pain accompanied by one-sided weakness, speech or vision problems, confusion, or loss of coordination

Chemical and Allergic Headaches

Chemical headaches are caused when chemicals from alcohol, pollution, cigarette smoke, poisons, medications, or other sources enter your blood. Chemical headaches are vascular headaches, which means they can cause blood flow changes that create pressure on blood vessels in the head. These vascular headaches will often throb with pain.

Allergies can also cause headaches. The pain from allergic headaches can be caused both by vascular changes and by pressure from congested sinuses.

The prevention and home treatment are the same as for tension headaches (see page 132) with the following additions:

- Identify and avoid the chemical or allergen that causes headaches.

- Breathe fresh air and drink lots of water to help flush the chemicals from your body.

Infection-Caused Headaches

Headaches can be caused by both viral and bacterial infections or inflammations. Headaches are common with colds and flu. The same home treatment as for tension headaches is advised (see page 132).

Sinusitis is a common cause of face and head pain (page 74). See also the home treatment sections for colds (page 68) and for flu (page 71).

The following problems are less common but more serious. Both require immediate attention from a physician.

Meningitis

Meningitis is a contagious infection of the membranes that cover the brain and spinal cord. Symptoms include fever, severe headache, vomiting, and stiff neck, followed by delirium and loss of consciousness. Immediate medical care and antibiotic treatment are required.

Tracking Your Headaches

If you suffer from recurring headaches of unknown cause, keep a record of all headache symptoms.

Record six things:

1. The date and time each started and stopped

2. The events that preceded the headache

3. The location of the pain and the direction that it radiates

4. The nature of the pain (steady, throbbing, burning, dull, etc.)

5. The severity of the pain

6. Other symptoms

This log will help your doctor if medical evaluation is needed.

Temporal Arteritis

Temporal arteritis (also known as cranial arteritis) is an inflammation and stiffening of the arteries in the head. The most common symptom is a continuous throbbing headache in the temples. The artery in the temple may be swollen and tender to touch. Symptoms include:

- One-sided headache

- Tenderness in the temple area

- Blurred vision

- Stiffness in the neck and shoulders

- Call your physician immediately if these symptoms develop.

Migraine Headaches

Migraine headaches, also called vascular headaches, are believed to be caused by changes in the flow of blood in the vessels of the brain. They are very painful, one-sided headaches that develop quickly and may recur daily or only once every few months. Because migraines often cause nausea, they are sometimes called "sick" headaches.

Some types of migraines are preceded by warning signs. The person may feel full of energy, sleepy, irritable, or depressed, and may see flashes or patterns of light. Dizziness and numbness on one side of the body may also precede a migraine.

Prevention

- Learn and practice relaxation techniques. See Chapter 21.

- Observe any patterns of diet or activities that seem to bring on migraines.

- Taking one baby aspirin (75 mg) per day can help some people prevent migraines. Take with milk to avoid stomach irritation. See aspirin precautions on page 336.

Home Treatment

- Lie down in a darkened room at the first sign of a migraine. Relax the entire body, starting with the forehead and eyes and working down to the toes. See page 302.

- Try the home treatment advice for tension headaches. See page 132.

- If a physician has prescribed medication for your migraines, take the recommended dose at the first sign that a migraine is coming.

When to Call a Health Professional

- If you suspect that your headaches are migraine headaches. Review page 10 before agreeing to any expensive tests.

- For information on relaxation and biofeedback techniques that may prevent migraines.

Migraine - continued

- For prescription medications which may help treat migraine headaches.

Tension Headaches

Most headaches are caused by muscle tension. Tension headaches are caused by the tightening of muscles in the back, shoulders, neck, and scalp. Both emotional stress and physical stress can be involved.

A tension headache may occur as pain all over the head or as a band of pressure around the head. The constant, dull pain usually occurs on both sides of the head. Other signs of stress-related headaches include:

- Sore neck and shoulders
- Fatigue and irritability
- Pain behind the eyes
- Difficulty falling asleep
- Inability to concentrate

Prevention

- Reduce physical stress:

  - Change positions often during desk work. Use good posture. See page 34.

  - Stretch for 30 seconds each hour.

  - Exercise regularly.

  - Learn to relax clenched teeth and jaws.

- Reduce emotional stress:

  - Practice relaxation techniques. See Chapter 21.

  - Calm yourself before and after stressful events.

  - Avoid stressful situations.

Home Treatment

- Aspirin, acetaminophen (Tylenol), or ibuprofen (Advil) may relieve a tension headache. Avoid frequent use. Take with milk or food to reduce stomach irritation.

- Calm yourself. Close your eyes, breathe deeply, and practice the relaxation response. See page 303.

- Lie down in a darkened room with a cool cloth on your forehead.

- Apply a heating pad to shoulders and neck.

- Try cold packs on the shoulders and neck. Some people find cold works better than heat.

- Massage the neck muscles.

- Brush your hair and scalp from front to back.

- Go for a walk. Exercise helps to relax tense muscles.

When to Call a Health Professional

- If unexplained headaches occur more than three times a week for three weeks in a row.

- If a headache comes on very suddenly.

- If a headache is very severe and cannot be relieved with home treatment.

- If headaches require use of pain relievers at least once a week for several weeks.

- If you need help discovering or eliminating the source of your tension headache.

Head Injury

Most bumps to the head are minor and heal as easily as bumps anywhere else. Head injuries that cause cuts often bleed very heavily because the blood vessels of the scalp are very close to the surface. This bleeding is very alarming, but does not always mean that the injury is severe.

However, head injuries that do not cause bleeding outside the skull may have caused life-threatening bleeding and swelling inside the skull. Anyone who has experienced a head injury should be watched carefully during the following 24 hours for signs of a severe head injury.

Prevention

- Don't ride a bike or motorcycle without a helmet.

- Don't dive into shallow water.

- See the Fall Prevention Checklist on page 24.

Home Treatment

- If there is bleeding, apply firm pressure directly over the wound with a clean cloth or bandage for ten minutes. If the blood soaks through, apply additional cloths over the first, without removing it.

- Apply ice or cold packs to reduce the swelling. A "goose egg" will likely appear anyway, but ice will help ease the pain.

- Watch for the following signs of a severe head injury immediately afterwards and every two hours thereafter for the next 24 hours:

  - Confusion. Ask the person his name, address, age, the date, etc.

  - Unusual pupil constriction. One pupil may constrict more or less than the other, or not at all.

  - Inability to move arms and legs on one side of the body, or slower movement on one side than the other.

  - Abnormally deep sleep, or difficulty waking up.

Head Injury - continued

- o Severe vomiting that continues after the first two to three hours.

- Continue observing the person every two hours during the night. Wake them up and check for any unusual symptoms. Call a physician immediately if you cannot wake the person or if they have any of the above symptoms.

- Check for injuries to other parts of the body, especially if the person has fallen. Often the excitement and alarm that accompanies a head injury will cause you to miss other injuries that also need attention.

When to Call a Health Professional

- If bleeding cannot be stopped and/or the wound looks like it will need stitches.

- If the person has lost consciousness at any time following the injury.

- If the person is very confused after the first few minutes.

- If there is nausea and vomiting after the first two to three hours or violent vomiting after the first 15 minutes. Limited nausea or vomiting at first is usually not serious.

- If the pupils do not constrict or do not constrict evenly.

- If there is double vision after the first minute.

- If a severe headache develops. "The worst headache I've ever had."

- If the person has any loss of memory for more than a minute.

- If there are seizures or convulsions.

- If there is weakness or numbness on one side.

If the brain was simple enough for us to understand it,
we would be too simple to understand it.
Ken Hill

9

Nervous System Problems

Senility. Losing your marbles. Dementia. These are words that many come to fear as they get older. Only rarely are such fears well-founded. Most people will retain mental vitality throughout their lives.

This chapter provides some basic information about delirium, dementia, Alzheimer's disease, and Parkinson's disease. The chapter works best if you use it to help someone else who is concerned about such problems. If you wonder whether one of these problems may be affecting you, ask someone you trust to help you with the information in this chapter. You will need an objective observer to ask certain questions and record your responses.

Delirium

Delirium is a sign that a physical illness is becoming more serious. Delirium requires prompt medical

attention. The symptoms of delirium are:

- Major problems with thinking--disjointed and fragmented thoughts

- Major problems with memory--reduced ability to learn new things and to remember recent events

- Major problems with perception--difficulty in distinguishing between dreams, hallucinations, and reality

- Very short attention span--low levels of alertness

- Disrupted sleep-wake cycle--daytime sleepiness and nighttime wakefulness

- Emotions of fear, apathy, rage, or depression

Delirium comes on quickly over a few hours or days, often overnight. The symptoms of delirium may come and go. The person may be

Delirium - continued

alert and coherent one minute; confused and drowsy the next. In most cases, it is completely gone in one to four weeks. Those who recover from the physical illness causing the delirium generally do not have continuing mental impairment.

Home Treatment

Following prompt medical treatment, these additional tips can contribute to recovery.

- Provide a good balanced diet.

- Eliminate possible vitamin deficiencies.

- Provide plenty of fluids.

- Try electrolyte drinks like Gatorade or the homemade electrolyte drink on page 333.

- Review medication dosages and schedules so that no more than the prescribed dose is given.

- Remove clutter from the room.

- Limit visitors to one or two at a time.

- Display a clock, calendar, and familiar photographs or objects.

- Provide good lighting during the day and a dimmed light at night.

When to Call a Health Professional

Delirium is a medical emergency. The underlying cause must be found and treated quickly. Call a health professional:

- Anytime the symptoms listed above cause you to suspect delirium.

- Anytime delirium symptoms occur with a fever or other signs of an acute illness.

- If the person's anger or agitation becomes unmanageable.

- When you do talk with a doctor, the focus will be to identify and treat the underlying illness that triggered the delirium. Present a detailed description of all the prescribed and over-the-counter medications the person has taken. Include the dosages taken and any possibilities of ingesting more medications than prescribed. Also discuss your home treatment plan as described above.

- Ask the physician if some medications can be discontinued or reduced until the cause of the delirium is found.

Dementia

The term "dementia" describes a condition of persistent mental deterioration. It involves memory, problem-solving, learning, and other mental functions. The mental problems are severe enough to interfere with daily living activities. Dementia, unlike delirium, usually comes on slowly over time and is relatively stable with little day-to-day fluctuation.

The general symptoms of dementia include:

- Short-term memory loss. (More than just an occasional forgetting of appointments, names, or where you put things.)

- Inability to complete moderately complex tasks (such as making soup from a packaged mix).

- Confusion

- Impaired judgment

- Getting lost in familiar places

- Paranoid, inappropriate, or bizarre behavior

The mental status exam on page 139 can also help to identify possible dementia problems. If mental impairment has come on suddenly, the problem may be delirium, not dementia. The table on page 141 helps to distinguish delirium from dementia.

There are over 100 separate health conditions that can cause or mimic dementia. Many are reversible with treatment. For others, no completely effective treatment is currently available.

Depression can often cause the symptoms of dementia. Think first of depression when you notice memory loss, confusion, or impaired judgment. Medical treatment is usually effective. See page 240 for information about depression.

Other common causes of dementia are:

- Alzheimer's disease (page 142)

- Vascular dementia or multi-infarct dementia, caused by many small strokes in the brain (page 143)

- Chronic infections

- Reactions to medications (page 145)

- Poor nutrition or poor hydration (too little water)

- Alcohol dementia

- Parkinson's disease (page 144)

- Hypothyroidism (page 127)

- Deficiency in vitamin B1 (thiamine) or vitamin B12

Home Treatment

The home management guidelines for dementia presented below can be helpful no matter what the cause of the problem.

- Simplify the daily routine with regular times for meals, baths, and a limited number of activities.

Dementia - continued

- Create a safe but interesting living environment. In addition to the safety checklists on pages 23-25, add the following:

  - Disconnect an electric stove when not in use.

  - Provide an ID bracelet.

  - Keep chemicals locked away.

  - Put bells on doors.

- Use written notes or instructions. Label objects.

- Provide regular stimulation of senses: touching, singing, exercising, hugging.

- Review with a physician or pharmacist all medications and dosages. See the list of medications that can contribute to mental confusion on page 145.

- Provide good nutrition and plenty of fluids.

- Use a non-confronting approach to behavior problems. Distraction often works best.

- Consider home treatment for depression (page 242).

- See also Chapter 24, Caregiver Secrets.

When to Call a Health Professional

- If the symptoms of dementia are interfering with the person's ability to carry on normal activities. See page 137.

- If the score of the mental status exam on pages 139-142 or other symptoms cause you to suspect dementia.

- If a person with diagnosed dementia becomes uncontrollably hostile or agitated.

- For a referral to a geriatric assessment team or a specialist in geriatrics. These professionals have special training to identify causes of dementia. Some causes of dementia are reversible and many symptoms can be effectively managed.

A Check-Up from the Neck Up (This is not a self-test; ask someone to help.)

To evaluate overall mental competence, use this three-part assessment.

Step 1: Mental Status Exam

Step 2: Distinguishing Between Delirium and Dementia

Step 3: Early Symptoms Review

Step 1: Mental Status Exam*

Adapted from Folstein, Folstein, and Mc-Hugh, 1975.

Orientation Questions

Read the questions out loud slowly and clearly. (Score 1 point for each correct answer.)

- What is the year?

- What is the season?

- What is the date?

- What is the day of the week?

- What is the month?

- What state are we in?

- What county are we in?

- What town are we in?

- What place are we in? (building, home, etc.)

- What room are we in?

Naming Questions

Name three objects (ball, flag, tree) one second apart. Ask the person to repeat all three. (Score 1 point for each correct answer.)

Calculation Questions

Have the person begin at 100 and count backward by 7's. Stop after 5 subtractions: 93, 86, 79, 72, 65. (Score 1 point for each correct answer.)

Or, if the person cannot or will not do the subtraction, ask him or her to spell the word "world" backwards: D L R O W. (Score 1 point for each correct letter.) Use the highest score of the subtraction and spelling questions in computing the total score.

Recall Questions

Ask the person to name the three objects that you named earlier: ball, flag, tree. (Score 1 point for each correct answer.)

Language Questions

- Show the person a pencil and ask him/her to name it. (1 point)

- Show the person a watch and ask him/her to name it. (1 point)

- Ask the person to repeat the following phrase: "No ifs, ands, or buts." (1 point)

- Give the person the following instructions: "Take a piece of paper in your right hand. Fold it in half and place it on the floor." (1 point for completing each step.)

- Write "Close your eyes" on a piece of paper and ask the person to read it and obey the instruction. (1 point)

- Tell the person to write a sentence. (1 point)

Check-Up - continued

- Ask the person to copy this design (1 point).

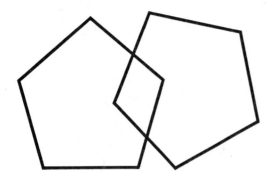

Interlocking shapes

Scoring

Total all the points. Often, a score of 23 or lower suggests a possible problem.

If the score is below 23, don't jump to conclusions. Poor hearing, a different first language, or a low level of education can also produce below-average scores. On the other hand, a high score does not guarantee there is no problem. Even so, most doctors will use a test like this as part of a mental assessment.

If the mental status exam causes you to suspect mental impairment, call your physician to discuss the need for a more complete assessment.

Step 2: Distinguishing Between Delirium and Dementia

Delirium and dementia are two different problems. You can use the chart on the next page to help understand the differences between them. Delirium and dementia can occur at the same time. Depression can also mimic the symptoms of delirium and dementia. See page 240.

If you suspect that the problem is delirium, call a physician immediately. Prompt diagnosis and treatment can be helpful. See more about delirium on page 135.

If you suspect that the problem is dementia, you may wish to read the section on dementia on page 136 before calling your doctor.

The causes of dementia are often difficult to identify and your input can be very helpful in the diagnosis.

Step 3: Early Symptoms Review

If the score on the mental status exam was above 23, but you still have concerns, continue with Step 3 of the assessment. This step will help identify any major or lasting changes that may be early signs of dementia. Consider the following examples:

Personality changes

- A normally social person becomes withdrawn.

- A person has unusual or wild mood swings.

Behavior changes

- A normally tidy person becomes messy.

- A person stops previous routines for no obvious reason.

- A person may become paranoid and suspicious of others.

Skill changes

- Loss of skill in balancing a checkbook

- Loss of skill in putting on makeup

- Loss of skill in cooking a favorite recipe

- Loss of ability to find previously familiar places

- Increasing and repeated confusion about times and dates

Delirium vs Dementia

Feature	Delirium*	Dementia
Onset	Rapid, often at night	Usually slow
Duration	Hours to weeks	Months to years
Course	Varies over 24 hours; some lucid intervals	Relatively stable, progessive over time
Awareness	Always impaired	Usually normal
Alertness	Varies up and down	Usually normal, in early stages
Orientation	Always impaired	May be intact
Memory	Sudden impairment	Gradual impairment
Thinking	Slow or fast, may be dreamlike	Poor in abstract thoughts
Sleep Cycle	Disrupted, drowsy during day; insomnia at night common	Fragmented sleep
Physical illness	Usually present, or medication problems	Often absent, unrelated, or medication problem
Perception	Illusions and hallucinations are common	Usually normal
For information	See page 135	See page 136

* Call a doctor immediately if delirium is suspected.

Check-Up - continued

- Increasing forgetfulness of where items are kept

Don't be overly concerned about minor changes in these areas. However, if the changes are major, unexplained, and causing increasing trouble, they can be clues that a more significant problem is developing. A review of the causes of dementia on page 137 may help you identify or rule out possible problems. Call a health professional if you suspect dementia.

Alzheimer's Disease

Alzheimer's disease is a condition that selectively damages the brain cells that affect memory, intelligence, judgment, and speech. The destruction of brain cells eventually leads to mental impairment, dementia, and death. There is currently no cure for Alzheimer's disease.

Alzheimer's disease develops very slowly. During the first two years, the only symptoms may be memory loss for recent events and occasional disorientation.

It may be difficult to distinguish these symptoms from the loss in the speed of memory recall that can be part of normal aging. As the disease progresses, however, memory loss continues and language and judgment become impaired. During this

Memory Loss Does Not Mean Alzheimer's

Alzheimer's disease causes disability in two groups of people: those who have the disease and those who fear they have it.

Many people have heard that an early sign of Alzheimer's disease is memory loss. So, when glasses are misplaced or names are forgotten, they worry that it is a sign of irreversible brain damage.

The facts are:

- Some slowing of memory response time is a normal consequence of aging, although not everyone is affected. See the discussion on memory and forgetfulness on page 248.

- Most older adults express some concerns about memory.

- Ninety percent of all people over age 65 do not have Alzheimer's disease.

- If memory loss does not interfere with your ability to carry on normal activities, you probably don't have Alzheimer's disease.

Don't let an occasional memory lapse cause you to forget to pursue a full life.

stage, the person may develop problems doing routine activities. In the final stage of the disease, the individual may become completely dependent upon others for all activities of daily living.

Prevention

Medical science is getting closer to finding the cause of Alzheimer's disease. However, until it does, prevention guidelines are limited.

Do your best to stay physically healthy and mentally active.

Home Treatment

The home treatment guidelines for Alzheimer's disease are the same as those for dementia on page 137.

In addition, you may wish to learn more about the illness by consulting Resources D1-2 on page 349. For more information, contact the Alzheimer's Association, 919 N. Michigan Ave., Suite 1000, Chicago, IL, 60611-1676, (800)272-3900.

When to Call a Health Professional

There are no definitive tests that will identify the early stages of Alzheimer's disease. Physicians rule out other causes of dementia before coming to a diagnosis of Alzheimer's.

The guidelines for when to call a doctor are the same as for dementia:

- If the score on the Mental Status Exam on page 139 is 23 or lower.

- If the symptoms of dementia are interfering with the person's ability to carry on normal activities. See page 137.

Multi-infarct Dementia

About 25 percent of all dementia is caused by blockages in tiny blood vessels in the brain. This is called multi-infarct dementia or vascular dementia. People with untreated diabetes or high blood pressure are at increased risk for multi-infarct dementia.

The symptoms of this kind of dementia vary depending on which area of the brain is affected. The person may successfully complete some sections of the mental status exam on page 139 but be unable to answer other sections.

Unlike Alzheimer's disease, which develops slowly, the onset of multi-infarct dementia is usually sudden. Symptoms develop in stages with some improvement between major declines in functioning. Depression and other symptoms of dementia listed on page 137 are often present.

Prevention

- Don't smoke.

- Keep blood pressure under control with both a healthy lifestyle and medication if necessary. See High Blood Pressure on page 86.

Multi-infarct Dementia - cont'd

- If you have high blood pressure or diabetes, and aspirin does not upset your stomach, ask your doctor about taking one regular aspirin daily.

The home treatment and advice for when to call a health professional are the same as for dementia on page 137.

Parkinson's Disease

Parkinson's disease is caused by a degeneration of the brain cells that produce dopamine. Dopamine is needed to transmit signals that control body movements. Parkinson's disease seldom strikes people younger than 50.

There is no known cure at this time. However, medication, diet, and exercise can relieve some symptoms. Treating Parkinson's in its early stages helps slow down the progress of the disease.

Early signs of Parkinson's include:

- Feeling slow and heavy

- Tiring easily

- Stiffness

- Slight hand tremor

These are vague symptoms which can go undiagnosed for a long time. You may pass them off as "just getting older."

As the disease advances, the symptoms become more pronounced:

- Shuffling walk and slow movements

- Tremor and shaking of the hands at rest

- Stooped posture, muscle rigidity, and stiffness

- Expressionless face

- Progressive dementia often develops

Prevention

Because the cause of Parkinson's disease is unknown, prevention guidelines are limited. Environmental toxins from agricultural chemicals may increase the risk, but are not the sole cause of the illness.

Home Treatment

- Provide good, well-balanced nutrition.

- Get regular exercise.

- Review home treatment for tremor on page 146.

- Consider home treatment guidelines for depression on page 242.

- Learn more about the illness by contacting the American Parkinson's Disease Association at (800) 223-2732 or the National Parkinson Foundation at (800) 327-4545.

Drugs That May Cause Mental Confusion*

Drug Type	Generic Name	Brand Name(s)
Major tranquilizers	chlorpromazine	Promapar, Sonazine, Thorazine
	haloperidol	Haldol, Halperon
Minor tranquilizers	diazepam	Valium, Valrelease, Vazepam
	chlordiazepoxide	Librium, Librax, Limbitrol, Lipoxide, Menrium
	alprazolam	Xanax
Sleeping tablets	lorazepam	Alzapam, Ativan
Parkinson's drugs	levodopa	Dopar, Larodopa, Sinemet
Antihistamines	promethazine	K-Phen, Pentazine, Phenergan, Prorex
Antidepressants	amitriptyline	Amitril, Elavil, Emitrip, Endep, Etrafon, Limbitrol, Triavil
	imipramine	Tofranil
Antiseizure drugs	phenytoin	Dilantin
Antihypertensives (high blood pressure drugs)	reserpine	Demi-Regroton, Diupres, Diutensen-R, Dureticyl, Enduronyl, Esidrix, Hydropres, Oreticyl, Rauzide, Regroton, Ser-Ap-Es, Serpalan, Unipres
	clonidine	Catapres
	methyldopa	Aldoclor, Aldomet, Aldoril
	propanolol	Inderal, Inderal-LA, Inderide, Inderide-LA, Ipran
	digoxin	Lanoxin
Painkillers	codeine	Tylenol-3, also in some over-the-counter cough medications, such as Robitussin-AC
	ibuprofen	Motrin, Advil, Nuprin
	naproxen	Anaprox, Naprosyn
Anticholinergic drugs	atropine	Donnatal
	dicyclomine	Bentyl
Antiulcer drugs	cimetidine	Tagamet
	ranitidine	Zantac

*This is not a complete list. If you have questions about any drugs and their effects, ask your doctor or pharmacist.

Parkinson's Disease - cont'd

When to Call a Health Professional

- If you suspect Parkinson's disease. New medications can provide effective treatment in many cases.

- Your doctor can also help you discover medications or other conditions that cause Parkinson-like symptoms.

Tremor

Tremor is an involuntary shaking or twitching movement that is repeated over and over. Tremor usually affects the hands and feet. Occasionally the head also shakes.

Tremors can be caused by many nervous system problems including Parkinson's disease, liver failure, alcoholism, and mercury or arsenic poisoning. Lithium, drugs taken for arrhythmias and hypertension, tricyclic antidepressants, and certain other medications can also cause tremor.

Family history plays a big role in essential tremor, which often begins before age 25. Mild symmetrical tremors of the head and both hands are often accepted as a normal consequence of aging, particularly in those over 70. Effective treatment is limited.

If you notice a tremor developing, carefully observe its nature and record its history before calling your health professional. If a cause is discovered, the disease will be treated rather than the tremor.

Home Treatment

- Stress reduction can help to reduce the severity of tremor. See Chapter 21.

- A physical change can reduce some tremors and restore more control to the hands.

  - Use a rigid brace across a joint.

  - Add a little weight to the hand.

  - Hold something in your hand.

- Convince yourself and those around you that although your hands may shake, your mind is steady.

When to Call a Health Professional

- If you suddenly develop a tremor or it suddenly becomes much worse.

You can observe a lot just by watching.
Yogi Berra (naturally)

10

Eyes and Seeing

By age fifty, most people have become aware of vision changes. Typical changes include:

- A gradual decline in the ability to see small print or focus on close objects (presbyopia)

- A decrease in the sharpness of vision

- The need for more light for certain activities, like reading or driving

- Some trouble distinguishing subtle color differences--blue may appear gray, for example

In addition to these normal changes, older eyes are also at greater risk for health problems. Minor irritations like dry eyes, excessive tearing, and "floaters" respond well to self-care and cause no permanent loss of vision. More serious problems, such as cataracts, glaucoma, and macular degeneration, require professional care to prevent vision loss or blindness.

This chapter will tell you what you can do to cope with normal changes in vision and what signs may indicate a more serious problem.

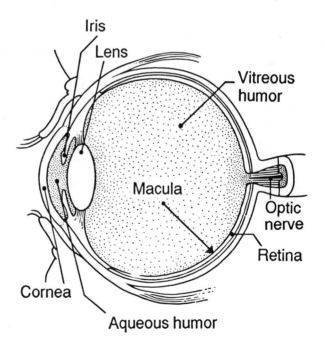

The Eye

The Aging Eyes

Common Eye Complaints

Presbyopia

Presbyopia (prez-bee-o-pea-ah), or farsightedness, is a condition that affects everyone sometime after age 40. As the eye ages, the lens becomes less flexible and can no longer easily focus on near objects or small print. You may find that you hold objects at arm's length to see them clearly. (People with presbyopia sometimes complain that they don't need glasses, they just need longer arms.)

Glasses or contact lenses correct this problem. If you already wear glasses, you may need bifocals. Avoid over-the-counter glasses; they will not take your individual vision needs into account.

Dry Eyes

Dry eyes occur when the tear glands are not producing enough tears. Your eyes will feel itchy, scratchy, and irritated. This may be associated with certain drugs (diuretics and antidepressants). Postmenopausal women are often susceptible to Sjogren's syndrome, which also causes dry eyes (see page 174).

Extreme dryness can damage eyes, so consult with your physician or eye specialist. "Artificial tears" or special eye drops can be prescribed to correct the problem. Some varieties are available over-the-counter.

Tearing

Excessive tears can be a sign of increased sensitivity to light or wind. Tearing may also mean an infection is present or that a tear duct is blocked.

If your eyes tear in reaction to strong light or wind, wear protective glasses. If they tear under other circumstances, call your eye specialist.

Floaters

Floaters are spots, specks, and lines that "float" across the field of vision. They are caused by stray cells or strands of tissue that float in the vitreous humor, the gel-like substance that fills the eyeball. Floaters can be annoying, but are not usually serious. However, if you notice a sudden increase in the number of floaters, or if they occur with flashes of light, call a health professional. This may be a sign of retinal detachment (see page 155).

Eye Emergencies

If you experience any of these problems, get immediate attention from an eye doctor:

- Severe eye pain

- Double vision

- Flashes or showers of light

- Sudden loss of vision, as if a curtain was pulled across your line of sight

---

Vision Protection Tips

Keep an eye on your sight throughout your life by following these general guidelines:

- Avoid overexposure to sunlight. Wear sunglasses that screen out ultraviolet (UV) rays. If you use tanning booths or sunlamps, wear opaque goggles.

- Wear goggles or protective glasses when you are exposed to strong chemicals, operating power tools, or playing racquet sports.

- Get periodic vision checkups: every two years if you wear glasses; every five years if you don't. More frequent checkups are recommended if you have a family history of eye disorders, diabetes, or a diagnosed vision disorder, such as glaucoma or cataracts.

- Always wash your hands before touching your eyes. Take care not to rub your eyes.

- Eat fruits and vegetables that contain beta carotene and/or vitamin C (cantaloupes, oranges, carrots). Some studies suggest that beta carotene delays or prevents cataracts.

- Avoid frequent use of over-the-counter eye drops. They may irritate the eye and cause allergic reactions.

- Keep your blood pressure under control. See page 86.

- If you have diabetes, follow the home treatment guidelines on page 121.

The Eye Specialists

Ophthalmologists are medical doctors (M.D.) or osteopathic doctors (D.O.) who are trained and licensed to provide total care of the eye. They can prescribe corrective lenses, diagnose and treat disorders of the eye, and perform surgery.

Optometrists (O.D.) perform eye examinations and prescribe corrective lenses. If they discover a medical problem, they will refer you to an ophthalmologist for diagnosis and treatment.

Opticians make eyeglasses and fill the prescriptions for corrective lenses.

Cataracts

Cataracts are thickened, hardened, and cloudy parts of the eye lens. The cloudy lens blocks or distorts light coming into the eye and blurs vision. Cataracts usually affect both eyes and develop at different rates. Some remain quite small and do not impair vision. When they become large enough to cause visual problems, the only effective treatment is surgery.

Cataracts - continued

Symptoms include painless blurring or fuzziness of vision, decreased night vision, and problems with glare. Double vision or spots may be seen and lights may have a halo around them. If left untreated, the lens will become milky and vision will be greatly reduced.

Cataracts are very common; 90 percent of people over age 75 have some type of cataract. In addition to normal changes in the aging eye, cataracts may be caused by overexposure to sunlight, a direct injury or blow to the eye, chemical burns, and electrical shocks. Smokers have increased risk. Native Americans, people with diabetes, and those who have taken steroids are at risk for cataracts at an early age.

In the past, surgery was delayed until the cataract had become "ripe" or very cloudy. Now, cataract surgery is recommended as soon as visual impairment becomes a problem. The success rate for the operation is estimated at 95 percent.

Prevention

- Avoid overexposure to sunlight. Use sunglasses that block ultraviolet (UV) light. Wearing a brimmed hat while outdoors helps, too.

Light Up Your Life

Improve the lighting in your home to compensate for any vision loss you may have. Good lighting will make your home safer and your activities more enjoyable.

- Increase lighting on steps and stairways.

- Use more than one light source in a room. It will help your eyes feel less tired.

- Use concentrated light for tasks that require near vision, such as reading or sewing.

- Cut down on glare. Use blinds or shades to cut down on direct sunlight. When you watch television, position the set so it doesn't reflect glare.

- Wear protective glasses or goggles when using strong chemicals or power tools, and when playing racquet sports.

- Eat foods high in beta carotene and/or vitamin C (cantaloupes, oranges, carrots, etc.) These foods seem to help prevent or delay cataracts.

- If you have diabetes, keep it under control. See page 121.

Home Treatment

Although you cannot stop or slow the progress of cataracts once they have developed, there are many things you can do to make the gradual changes in your vision easier to live with.

- Make sure you have plenty of light indoors. Standard 60 to 100 watt light bulbs seem to work best for most people; fluorescent lights are less helpful. Use table or floor lamps for reading or other close work.

- When outdoors, wear sunglasses with yellow-tinted lenses, which will help to reduce glare. A large-brimmed hat or visor will help, also. However, sunglasses do not help everyone, so experiment before you buy an expensive pair.

- When you watch television, don't have a light on between you and the screen. It will produce glare.

- Try large-print books and newspapers. Magnifying glasses may help you read some things, but only if the type is very clear. Magnified blurry print will be larger, but will still be blurry.

- For more information on cataracts and other vision problems, contact The Lighthouse, 800 Second Avenue, New York, NY 10017, (212) 808-0077.

When to Call a Health Professional

- To schedule periodic eye exams. See page 26 for recommended frequency.

- If you are bothered by blurred or fuzzy vision.

- If your night vision is impaired.

Chemicals in the Eye

Chemical burns to the eye occur when something caustic, such as window-cleaning fluid, gasoline, or turpentine splashes into it. The eye appears red and watery. If the damage is severe, the eye will appear whitish.

Prevention

- Wear protective goggles or glasses when working with chemicals.

Home Treatment

Immediately flush the eye with tap water to dilute the chemical. Put your face into a sink or dish pan filled with water. Open and close your eyes rapidly. Keep it up until the eye stops hurting. A squirt bottle will also work well.

Chemicals in the Eye - cont'd

> ### Blood in the Eye
>
> Sometimes, blood vessels in the whites of the eyes break and cause a red spot or speck on the eye. This is called a subconjunctival hemorrhage. The blood in the eye may look alarming, especially if the spot is large. It is usually not a cause for concern, and will clear up in two to three weeks.
>
> However, if your eye is bloody and painful, or if the bleeding followed a blow to the eye, call a health professional. Also call if bleeding in the eye occurs often, or if you are taking medication to thin your blood.

When to Call a Health Professional

- After flushing the eye, go immediately to an emergency center if there is major exposure to a strong acid, such as battery acid, or to a caustic substance such as lye or Drano.

- If the eye still hurts after 20 minutes of home treatment.

- If the eye appears damaged. Symptoms include:

  - Persistent redness

  - Discharge

  - Watering

  - Any visual disturbance such as double vision, blurring, or sensitivity to light

  - Colored part of the eye appears white

Conjunctivitis

Conjunctivitis, or "pink eye," is an inflammation of the conjunctiva, the delicate membrane that lines the inside of the eyelid and the surface of the eye. It can be caused by bacteria, viruses, allergies, air pollution, or other irritants.

The symptoms are redness in the whites of the eyes, red and swollen eyelids, lots of tears, and a scratchy, sandy feeling in the eyes. There may be a discharge that causes the eyelids to stick together during sleep.

Most cases of conjunctivitis will clear up spontaneously, or your doctor can prescribe antibiotic eye drops. Good home care will speed healing and bring relief.

Prevention

- Wash your hands thoroughly after treating a person with pink eye.

- Avoid eye-rubbing as it can transfer the condition from one eye to the other.

- Do not share towels, handkerchiefs, or washcloths with an infected person.

- If an irritant gets into the eye, immediately flush it with tap water. The simplest method is to fill a sink with cool water, dunk the face, and blink several times under water.

Home Treatment

- Apply cold compresses every three hours to relieve itching.

- Gently wipe the eye with moist cotton or a clean washcloth and water to remove encrusted matter.

- If eye drops are prescribed, insert in the following manner:

  - Pull the lower lid down with two fingers to create a little pouch.

  - Put the drops there.

  - Close the eye to let the drops move around.

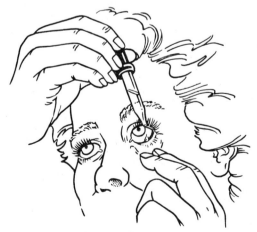

Inserting Eye Drops

Be sure the dropper is clean and does not touch any surface. Eye drops are washed out by normal tearing, so they will need to be replaced frequently, usually every four hours.

When to Call a Health Professional

- If the eye is red and there is a thick, greenish-yellow discharge.

- If there is distinct pain in the eye rather than irritation.

- If vision is distorted or blurred.

- If the problem is very bothersome, getting worse, or recurring.

- If there is an abnormal difference in the size of the pupils. A constricted pupil may indicate an infection of the iris, which needs medical attention.

- If the problem continues for more than a week.

Glaucoma

Glaucoma is an eye disorder caused by too much pressure within the eyeball. This pressure (ocular hypertension) builds up when the fluid (aqueous humor) in the chamber between the lens and the cornea is unable to drain normally. If the pressure is not relieved, it may eventually cause damage to the retina and optic

Glaucoma - continued

nerve and result in blindness. Untreated glaucoma is one of the leading causes of blindness in older adults.

Glaucoma is normally painless and can develop slowly over several years without being detected. Warning signals include blurred vision, reduced side vision ("tunnel vision"), and halos around lights.

A rare form of the disorder, called closed-angle glaucoma, comes on quite suddenly and can lead to permanent damage in a matter of 24 hours. This condition is marked by severe pain in the eye, blurred vision, and a reddened eyeball. This is a medical emergency and must be attended to at once.

People who are at increased risk for developing glaucoma include:

- Those with a family history of the disorder

- Those who are nearsighted or have diabetes

- Those who take corticosteroid drugs

- African-Americans

Prevention

The goal is to detect glaucoma before vision loss occurs. People aged 50 to 64 are advised to have a glaucoma test every five years. If you are at high risk for glaucoma, schedule an exam every year after age 50.

Home Treatment

Regular and consistent use of medications prescribed for glaucoma is important. Follow your doctor's guidelines.

When to Call a Health Professional

- If vision is blurred or if you see halos around lights.

- If there is severe pain in the eye or the white of the eye is reddened.

Macular Degeneration

Macular degeneration is the leading cause of blindness for those over age 50. It is caused by damage or breakdown of the macula, the part of the retina that provides clear, sharp central vision. It may occur in one or both eyes.

Early signs of macular problems include distortion in vertical lines (for example, a telephone pole will appear to have a "blip" in it), blurred or cloudy vision, a dark or blind spot at the center of vision, and dimmed color vision. Eventually, central vision in the affected eye will be lost; peripheral, or side, vision will not be affected.

If you notice these symptoms, see your ophthalmologist as soon as possible. Depending upon the type of macular degeneration you have, laser-beam therapy may slow the progress of the degeneration. To be effective, therapy must be applied within a matter of days after symptoms appear. Zinc supplements have also been shown to have some positive effect. Talk with your ophthalmologist.

Prevention

Since early detection and immediate action are so crucial, the goal of prevention is to be alert for problems. Do this simple self-test regularly:

- Cover one eye.

- Focus on a straight line, such as a door frame or telephone pole. Check for any wavy lines.

- Repeat with the other eye.

The Amsler Grid (see illustration) is a simple test to check for macular problems. Cover one eye and look at the dot in the center of the grid.

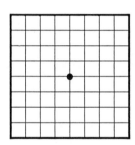

Amsler Grid

If lines around the dot look wavy or distorted, you may have a macular problem.

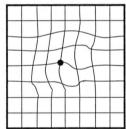

Home Treatment

People with macular degeneration can benefit from special devices that help them make the most of side vision. Talk with your ophthalmologist.

When to Call a Health Professional

- If vision is blurry while reading or doing close-up work, such as sewing.

- If straight lines appear wavy.

- If a dark or blind spot appears at the center of vision.

- If colors seem dim.

Other Retinal Disorders

Detached Retina

Most retinal detachments are caused by small tears or holes in the retina. People at risk for detached retinas include older adults, people who are nearsighted, and those with a family history of retinal detachments. A blow to the head or eye may also cause the retina to detach.

Retinal Disorders - continued

The sudden appearance of spots or flashes of light, or dark shadows in your field of vision may indicate a tear in the retina. Have these symptoms checked out by an eye doctor. Prompt treatment can save your eyesight.

Diabetic Retinopathy

This is a possible complication of diabetes. It occurs when the retina does not get enough oxygen because of damage to the blood vessels that normally nourish it. Symptoms include clouding of vision and seeing spots. People with diabetes need yearly eye checkups so the condition may be diagnosed early. Appropriate treatment can prevent vision loss.

Objects in the Eye

When something gets in your eye that tears cannot remove, try not to rub it; you could scratch the cornea.

Prevention

Always wear protective goggles or glasses when operating power tools.

Home Treatment

- First, wash your hands.

- If the object is in the side of the eye or by the lower lid, moisten the tip of a twisted piece of tissue and touch the speck with the end. The debris should cling to the tissue.

- You may also try this simple method: gently grasp the lashes of your upper lid and pull the lid down over the lower lashes. Hold for a few seconds and release. Sometimes this will remove small particles.

- Gently wash the eye with cool water; an eyedropper helps.

- Never use tweezers, toothpicks, or other hard items to remove any object. Damage may result.

When to Call a Health Professional

- If the object is on the eyeball rather than on the eyelid. You could damage the eye if the object severely scratches the eyeball. This is especially true if an object has penetrated the eyeball.

- If you cannot remove the object yourself.

- If the object has scratched the cornea. Although most corneal scratches are minor and self-healing, pain that persists after the object is removed should be checked out.

Styes

A sty is an infection of the eyelash root (follicle) that appears as a small, red bump, much like a pimple. It usually comes to a head and breaks after a few days. Most styes respond to home treatment and clear up in a week or so.

Prevention

Styes are easily passed among family members. If you have a sty, wash your hands often so you don't spread the infection.

Home Treatment

• Do not rub the eye.

• Apply warm, moist compresses for 10 minutes three times a day until the sty comes to a point and drains. Do not squeeze a sty.

• Use clean washcloths, towels, and pillowcases every day.

When to Call a Health Professional

• If there is no improvement after two days of home treatment.

• If the sty interferes with vision.

• If many styes appear at once or if styes occur often.

Help for Vision Problems

The National Eye Care Project is a public service program sponsored by the Foundation of the American Academy of Ophthalmology and volunteer ophthalmologists. It provides medical and surgical eye care for disadvantaged older adults who are:

• 65 or older

• US citizens or legal residents

• Without access to an ophthalmologist

Call toll-free for help
• **1-800-222-EYES**

To get a free catalog of low-vision aid devices, write to: American Foundation for the Blind, Consumer Products Division, 15 West 16th Street, New York, NY 10011, (800)232-5463 or (212)620-2147 for NY residents.

*The older I grow,
the more I listen to people who don't say much.*
Germain Glidden

11

Ears and Hearing

The human ear is a delicate organ designed to channel and modify sound waves. Sound waves enter the ear and cause the eardrum to vibrate, setting in motion the tiny bones of the middle ear: the hammer, anvil, and stirrup. These bones transfer sounds to the structures of the inner ear--the cochlea and auditory nerve. The cochlea contains tiny hairs that convert sounds to nerve impulses that are transmitted to the brain by the auditory nerve.

As we get older, a number of changes within the ear can affect how well we hear. For example, the tiny hairs in the cochlea begin to deteriorate and do not conduct the sound vibrations as well. This breakdown is probably due to lifelong exposure to noise.

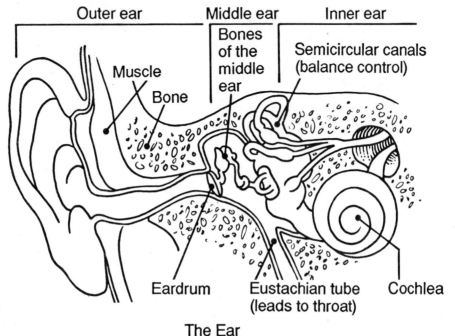

The Ear

It is impossible to go back in time and undo noise damage, but there is still plenty you can do to get the most out of your hearing.

This chapter will tell you how to protect your hearing and what you can do to cope with hearing losses and other ear problems.

Ear Infections

Ear infections are usually caused by bacteria and require antibiotic treatment. Symptoms of a bacterial ear infection may include pain, dizziness, ringing or fullness in the ear, hearing loss, fever, headache, and runny nose.

Prevention

- Treat a cold rapidly, especially if you have frequent ear infections. See page 68.

- Blow your nose gently, keeping your mouth open to avoid forcing fluid into the eustachian tubes.

Home Treatment

- Use a warm washcloth or heating pad to apply heat to the ear. This will ease pain.

- Rest. Let your energy go to fighting the infection.

- Drink plenty of clear liquids.

- Take aspirin or acetaminophen to help relieve earache pain. (Do not give aspirin to a child unless it has been prescribed by a physician.)

- Take the full course of antibiotics, if prescribed. Call if you have any reaction to the drug.

When to Call a Health Professional

- If any earache lasts over one hour and is accompanied by acute pain. If the pain is severe at night, call the next morning, even if the pain has stopped. The infection may still be present.

- If patient cannot touch chin to chest without pain. This may be a sign of meningitis, an inflammation of the membrane that covers the brain, especially if the person also has a fever, severe headache, and is confused or drowsy.

- If you suspect an eardrum rupture. Look for a white or yellow discharge from the ear.

- If there is no improvement after two to three days of antibiotics.

Ear Wax

Ear wax is a protective secretion, similar to mucus or tears, that filters dust and keeps the ears clean. Normally, ear wax is liquid, self-draining, and does not cause problems. Occasionally, the wax will build up, harden, and cause some hearing loss.

Once ear wax has hardened, poking at the wax with cotton swabs, fingers, or other objects will only pack the wax more tightly against the eardrum. Professional help is needed to remove tightly packed wax. You can handle most ear wax problems by avoiding cotton swabs and following the home treatment tips below.

Home Treatment

- Lie down with a warm damp cloth under the affected ear. This should cause the wax to soften and drain out.

- Warm water helps loosen wax. Stand under a warm shower with your ear tilted toward the shower-head or wash wax out with an ear syringe and warm water. (Cold water may make you dizzy. Use very gentle force.) Do not use this technique if there is a discharge from the ear or if you suspect the eardrum is ruptured.

- If the warm cloth and shower do not work, use an over-the-counter wax softener each night for three to four nights.

When to Call a Health Professional

- If the above procedures do not work and the wax build-up is hard, dry, and compacted.

- If you suspect that ear wax is causing a hearing problem.

- If soreness or bleeding from your ear occurs.

The Hearing Specialists

Otologists or otolaryngologists are medical doctors (M.D.) or doctors of osteopathy (D.O.) with extensive training in ear and hearing problems. They can diagnose and treat hearing disorders and perform surgery.

Audiologists help people identify and manage hearing problems. They are licensed to conduct hearing tests and dispense hearing aids. They do not prescribe drugs or perform surgery.

Hearing aid specialists conduct evaluations for the purpose of selling and fitting hearing aids. They are generally not licensed and may or may not have adequate training for hearing evaluations.

Hearing Loss

Hearing loss is one of the most common conditions affecting people over 50. There are three types of hearing loss: conductive, sensorineural, and central deafness.

Conductive hearing loss results from the blockage or interference of sound to the inner ear. The most common

Hearing Loss - continued

cause is packed ear wax in the ear canal. This is easily remedied (see page 160). Infection, abnormal bone growth, and excess fluid in the ear are other causes.

People with conductive hearing loss often complain that their own voice sounds loud while other voices sound muffled. There may be a low level of tinnitus, or ringing in the ear. Conductive hearing loss, depending on the underlying problem, is usually treated by ear-flushing, medicines, or surgery.

Most hearing loss is caused by problems in the inner ear or acoustic nerve. This is called sensorineural hearing loss. The damage to the inner ear can be the result of changes that come with age, environmental noise, and some medications, specifically aspirin.

People with sensorineural hearing loss generally do not suffer from total deafness. They may have trouble understanding the speech of others while being very sensitive to loud sounds. The person may hear ringing, hissing, or clicking noises.

Central deafness is quite rare. It is caused by damage to the hearing centers in the brain. Stroke, lengthy high fever, or a blow to the head may cause central deafness. The person with central deafness can hear normally but has difficulty understanding what is heard.

Caregiver Tips: Living with a Hearing-Impaired Person

- Speak to the person at a distance of three to six feet. Make sure that your face, mouth, and gestures can be seen clearly. Arrange furniture so everyone is completely visible.

- Avoid speaking directly into the person's ear. Visual clues will be missed.

- Speak slightly louder than normal, but do not shout. Speak slowly.

- Cut down on background noise. Turn down the television or radio. Ask for quiet sections in restaurants.

- If a particular phrase or word is misunderstood, find another way of saying it. Avoid repeating the same words over and over.

- If the subject is changed, tell the person, "We are talking about ____ now."

- Treat the hearing-impaired person with respect and consideration. Involve the person in discussions, especially about him or her. Do what you can to ease feelings of isolation.

Facts About Hearing Aids

Elements and Models

- Microphone to pick up the sound
- Amplifier to make it louder
- Receiver to transmit the sound to the ear
- Battery for power
- Volume control to regulate sound level
- Ear mold to keep the aid in place
- Canal aid which fits directly into the ear
- Style that fits behind the ear
- Hearing aids that fit into the frames of eyeglasses
- Body aid which is carried in a pocket with wires leading up to the ear mold

Questions to Ask Before You Buy

- What kind of hearing aid will best suit my needs?
- How much does each hearing aid cost? The price will depend on the style of hearing aid, the amount of power needed, the manufacturer's brand, and from whom you buy the aid.
- Will Medicare/Medicaid and private health insurance pick up any of the costs? Medicare may pay for some of the fitting costs. Your insurance or health plan coverage may also pay some of the costs.
- What does the cost of the hearing aid cover? Check to see if special services, follow-up visits, and adjustments are covered. Also ask about warranties.
- Does the audiologist/hearing aid specialist offer a 30-day trial period before the purchase becomes final?

Considerations

- Not all hearing loss can be corrected with a hearing aid; it depends on the underlying cause of the loss.
- Hearing aids work by making sounds louder. They do not restore normal hearing. As the sound is intensified, it also becomes distorted.
- It takes time and practice to get used to a hearing aid; many people find them difficult to adjust to. Wear your hearing aid every day and gradually accustom yourself to the way it works.

Hearing Loss - continued

Prevention

- Wear ear plugs when exposed to loud noise, or avoid it if possible.

- Keep your ears clean and periodically check for wax buildup. See page 160.

- Do not use cotton swabs or other objects to clean your ears. They may damage the ear canal or drum and may force wax deep into the ear. The same old advice still applies: Never stick anything smaller than your elbow in your ear.

- Keep circulatory problems, such as heart disease, high blood pressure, and diabetes under control. Some hearing loss may be the result of impaired circulation.

- Be aware of medication side effects on hearing. Antibiotics (gentamicin), blood pressure medicine (diuretics such as Lasix), ibuprofen, and large doses of aspirin (8 to 12 pills per day) are linked to hearing impairment.

Home Assessment

To check your hearing, you can perform a few simple tests:

The Clock Test

- Have a friend hold a clock out of sight some distance from one side of your head.

- Have the friend move slowly closer. Tell him when the ticking is first heard.

- Repeat for the other ear. You should hear the sound about the same distance away from each ear.

- Test your friend's hearing in the same way to see if he can hear the clock from much farther away than you can. (Be sure to ask a friend whose hearing is good!)

The Radio Test

- Have someone adjust the volume on a radio so it is pleasing to that person. Can you hear it well or do you have to strain?

The Telephone Test

- When you talk on the telephone, switch the phone from ear to ear to hear if the sound is the same. Although the hearing loss of aging usually affects both ears, it is possible that only one ear is affected.

When to Call a Health Professional

- Between the ages of 50 and 64, hearing exams are recommended every 10 years. After age 65, increase to every five years. Have exams more frequently if hearing problems exist.

- If hearing loss develops suddenly (within a matter of days or weeks).

- If you experience ringing in the ear, dizziness, ear pain, headache, or fluid loss from the ear.

- To consider a hearing aid. Make an appointment with a hearing specialist if you find:

  - You often ask people to repeat themselves.

  - You cannot hear soft sounds, such as a dripping faucet, or high-pitched sounds.

  - You continuously hear a ringing or hissing background noise.

  - You have difficulty understanding words.

  - You have difficulty hearing when someone speaks in a whisper.

  - Your personal and social life are hampered by a hearing problem.

Tinnitus (Ringing Ears)

Almost everyone has experienced an occasional ringing sound in the ears. Usually the sound passes within a few moments. When the ringing (or possibly hissing, buzzing, humming, or tinkling) becomes persistent, you may have tinnitus.

Tinnitus is most commonly caused by permanent nerve damage to the inner ear from prolonged exposure to loud noise. Other, more treatable causes include excess ear wax, ear infections, and medications (especially antibiotics and large amounts of aspirin). Tinnitus may also be caused by tumors, head injuries, and excessive use of alcohol.

Meniere's Disease

Meniere's disease is characterized by attacks of vertigo, tinnitus, nausea and vomiting, and hearing loss. The person may also be very sensitive to loud noises.

Meniere's disease is caused by an accumulation of fluid in the inner ear. The attacks can last several minutes or hours and come as frequently as once a week or as seldom as once a year.

If you have been diagnosed with Meniere's disease, these measures may help ease symptoms:

- Restrict salt, caffeine, and alcohol.

- Stop smoking.

- Ease stress with relaxation techniques. Attacks often come during periods of emotional upset. See Chapter 21.

Tinnitus - continued

Prevention

- Wear ear plugs when exposed to loud noises, such as power tools, gunshots, jet engines, or industrial machinery.

- Limit your aspirin use. See aspirin precautions on page 336.

Home Treatment

Tinnitus must be treated by a health professional. However, there are steps you can take to ease symptoms:

- Reduce your use of alcohol, caffeine, nicotine, and aspirin.

- Try to relax. Stressful situations seem to aggravate tinnitus. See pages 300-304 for some simple relaxation techniques.

- Find emotional support; tinnitus can be difficult to deal with. The American Tinnitus Association is a helpful support group. Write P.O. Box 5, Portland, OR 97207 (enclose a self-addressed stamped envelope).

When to Call a Health Professional

- If the noises you hear in your ear are persistent, loud, and interfere with your daily activities or sleep.

- If you experience some hearing loss along with the tinnitus.

- If you experience vertigo, a sensation of dizziness combined with a feeling of spinning. See below.

- If nausea and vomiting accompany tinnitus.

- To discuss medical treatment to relieve tinnitus.

Vertigo/Dizziness

Inner ear disorders may lead to vertigo, a feeling of extreme dizziness accompanied by a sensation of movement or spinning. (The key difference between dizziness and vertigo is the perception of the spinning motion.) Nausea and vomiting may also go along with vertigo.

Older adults are prone to attacks of vertigo. One of the most common forms is benign positional vertigo, which comes on suddenly when you stand up quickly, lean your head back to look up at something, or when you turn over in bed. Vertigo may also be caused by ear infections and ear wax build-up. It can be a side effect of medications, particularly drugs for high blood pressure. Other underlying problems that can contribute to vertigo are heart disease, high blood pressure, anemia, and diabetes.

Dizziness or fainting may occur when there is a change in blood flow to the brain. Dizziness can be caused by medications, sudden emotional stress, or injury. It is also common when a person who has a cold or the flu, or who takes high blood pressure medications, suddenly sits up or stands up.

Prevention

- Do two minutes of exercise before getting out of bed.

- Get up from bed or from a chair slowly. Sit on the edge of the bed for a few minutes before standing.

Home Treatment

During a bout of vertigo or dizziness, you are at risk for injury resulting from a fall or other mishap. Lie down or sit until the sensation passes.

When to Call a Health Professional

- If you suspect vertigo. Your doctor will help determine the cause. Tell your doctor about any medications you are taking.

- If you completely lose consciousness.

- If dizziness is accompanied by a headache, loss of hearing, weakness in the arms or legs, blurred vision, or numbness in any part of the body.

- If dizziness may be caused by medications.

- If dizziness continues for over two to three days, or if you are concerned that fainting may cause injury.

Help for Hearing Problems

- SHHH (Self Help for Hard of Hearing People, Inc.) 7800 Wisconsin Avenue, Bethesda, MD 20814

  - (301) 657-2248 (Voice)

  - (301) 657-2249 (TDD)

- American Speech-Language-Hearing Association

  - (800) 638-8255

- For free booklets on hearing problems or a free over-the-phone hearing test, call

  - (800) 222-EARS

  - in Pennsylvania, call (800) 345-EARS

- The Better Hearing Institute provides information on hearing protection and deafness prevention. M-F 9AM to 5PM EST.

  - (800) EAR-WELL

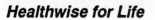

Be true to your teeth or your teeth will be false to you.
Dental Proverb

12

Mouth, Throat, and Dental Problems

Just like the rest of the body, your mouth and throat are affected by advancing age. Typical changes include:

- A difference in your sense of taste. Age-related changes, dentures, and medications can alter your sense of taste.

- Variations in your voice. See page 176 on voice changes with age.

- Tooth decay in "new" places. As gums recede, tooth roots are exposed and become more vulnerable to cavities. Decay around the edges of fillings is also common in older adults. See page 172 for prevention tips.

- Increased risk of gum disease. See page 172.

- Dentures and bridge work are more commonly found in older adults. See page 173 for helpful hints.

- Reduced saliva flow results in a dry mouth. See page 174 for what to do.

Understanding what changes are in store, and what you can do about them, is important to maintaining good oral health. This chapter also covers those irritations to your mouth and throat, such as canker sores, cold sores, and sore throats, that know no age limits.

Canker Sores

Canker sores are painful little blisters on the inner membranes of the mouth and cheek that break and leave open sores. There are many possible causes of canker sores. Injury to the inside of the mouth, genetic predisposition, female hormones, and stress all seem to play a role. The sores usually heal by themselves in about ten days.

Canker Sores - continued

Prevention

- Avoid injury to the inside of your mouth:

  ○ Chew food slowly and carefully.

  ○ Use a soft-bristle toothbrush and brush your teeth thoroughly but gently.

Home Treatment

- Avoid eating spicy and salty foods, and citrus fruits.

- Apply an oral paste, like Orabase, to the canker sore. It will stick to the sore and protect it, ease pain, and speed healing.

- Try an antihistamine mouthwash, such as Benadryl.

- A thin paste of baking soda and water may bring relief.

When to Call a Health Professional

- If mouth sores developed after starting a medication.

- If a canker sore, or any sore, does not heal after 14 days.

- If a sore is very painful or comes back frequently.

- If white spots that are not canker sores appear in the mouth and do not heal within two to three weeks.

Oral Cancer

Risk Factors

- Cigarette, cigar, or pipe smoking

- Use of chewing tobacco

- Excessive use of alcohol

When to Call a Health Professional

- If a mouth or lip sore bleeds easily and doesn't heal within two to three weeks.

- If a lump or thickening appears in the mouth, neck, lips, or tongue.

- If a red or white scaly patch appears on the lips or inside the mouth.

- If you have unexplained difficulty in chewing, swallowing, or moving the tongue or jaw.

Cold Sores (Fever Blisters)

Cold sores, or fever blisters, are caused by a herpes virus. They are small red blisters that have a dry ring around a moist center. Cold sores appear outside the mouth, unlike canker sores, which appear inside the mouth.

Cold sores may appear after colds, fevers, or exposure to the sun. They are contagious; don't expose others. Avoid sharing drinking glasses and eating utensils, and kissing while you have a cold sore.

Home Treatment

- Be patient. Cold sores usually go away within seven to ten days.

- Blistex or Campho-Phenique may ease the pain. Don't share with others.

- Cornstarch may be soothing. Apply in a paste made with a little water.

When to Call a Health Professional

- If sores last longer than two weeks.

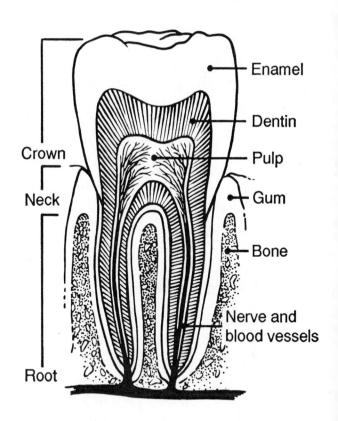

The Tooth

Dental Problems

Dental disease is a preventable health problem. You can keep all of your teeth by practicing good home care and having regular professional check-ups. Be on the lookout for tooth decay and gum disease--both can appear as the result of bacterial plaque.

Plaque and Tooth Decay
Bacteria are always present in the mouth. When they are undisturbed by brushing and flossing, bacteria stick to the teeth and multiply into larger and larger colonies called plaque. It appears as a sticky, color-less film on your teeth.

This sticky plaque damages teeth in two ways. First, food particles, especially refined sugars, stick to it. The plaque uses that food to grow more bacteria and to produce acid. Second, the plaque holds the acid against the tooth surface and prevents saliva and water from mixing with it. Left alone, the acid will eventually eat through the tooth enamel, causing tooth decay.

If you eat only at meal times, it takes about 24 hours for bacteria and acid to harm your teeth. This is enough time for you to brush the plaque off and to wash away the acid. If you eat

Dental Problems - continued

a lot of between-meal snacks, plaque can build up more quickly. Tooth-brushing will be required more frequently.

Plaque and Periodontal (Gum) Disease

Periodontal disease, an inflammation around the gums and in the bone sup-porting the gums, is the primary cause of tooth loss in older adults It is caused by bacterial plaque that builds up and sticks to the teeth.

The first stage of the disease, called gingivitis, is marked by swollen, bleeding gums and bad breath. This stage is painless and, unfortunately, many people do not seek treatment.

As the disease progresses, the supporting bones and ligaments are affected. The teeth move apart from each other, creating gaps between them. Eventually the teeth fall out.

People with diabetes and those who smoke or chew tobacco are at increased risk. However, everyone is at risk; some estimates indicate that 75 percent to 80 percent of Americans have some form of periodontal disease.

Faithful home care and regular visits to the dentist can prevent tooth decay and periodontal disease.

Prevention

- Brush and floss properly to remove plaque. A thorough job once a day is better than two or

Get a Hold of Your Toothbrush

If you have difficulty brushing your teeth because your hands are stiff, painful, or weak, consider these simple solutions:

- Enlarge the brush handle by wrapping a sponge, elastic bandage, or adhesive tape around it. You might also push the handle through a rubber ball.

- Lengthen the handle by taping popsicle sticks or tongue depressors to it.

- Use an electric toothbrush.

There are also specially designed toothbrushes, toothpaste dispensers, and floss holders. See Resource H1 on page 350.

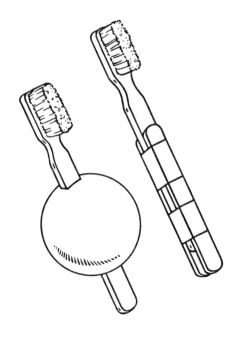

Adapted Toothbrushes

three quick brushings. Clean every part of every tooth.

- Use fluoride toothpaste or mouth rinses. Fluoride is a mineral that strengthens tooth enamel and reduces the harmful effects of plaque.

- Eat crunchy foods that naturally clean the teeth (apples, lettuce, and other raw vegetables), and foods with ample vitamin C, like citrus fruits and broccoli.

- Have your teeth checked and cleaned at least twice a year by a dentist or dental hygienist.

Home Treatment

- Occasional bleeding when you brush or floss is an early sign that gum disease is present. However, with good care, it won't take too long to get back to normal. Brush and floss your teeth every day, and follow the prevention guidelines.

When to Call a Health Professional

- For regular cleanings and exams. Every six months is recommended.

- If your gums bleed when you push on them or bleed often when you brush your teeth.

- If teeth are loose or moving apart.

- If there are changes in the way your teeth fit together when you bite or in the way partial dentures fit.

- If gums are very red, swollen, or tender, or if pus is present.

Denture Care

- Clean your dentures every day with a brush and a denture cleaner such as Polident.

- Keep the dentures in lukewarm water or a denture-cleansing liquid overnight.

- Examine your gums daily before putting in your dentures. Let red, swollen gums heal before wearing your dentures again. If the redness does not go away in a few days, call your dentist. White patches on the inside of the cheeks could also indicate poorly fitting dentures.

- Don't put up with dentures that are too big, click during eating, or feel uncomfortable. Dentures take some time to get used to, but if they are still giving you trouble after the first few weeks, consult your dentist about a refitting.

Dental Problems - continued

- If you have a toothache. Tooth- aches are caused when the inside of the tooth, the dentin, is ex- posed. The pain may go away tem- porarily, but the problem will not. Take aspirin or acetaminophen (Tylenol) for pain relief until you can get an appointment. A cold pack on the jaw may also help.

Dry Mouth

Many older adults experience dry mouth (xerostomia). It can be caused by:

- Breathing through the mouth in dry environments

- Diabetes

- Many common drugs, particularly diuretics and antihistamines

- Not drinking enough water throughout the day

- Gum disease

- Radiation therapy to the head or neck

- Autoimmune diseases such as rheumatoid arthritis and Sjogren's syndrome (see box at right)

Chronic lack of saliva can cause serious oral problems, such as tooth decay and bacterial infections.

Prevention

- Humidify your home, especially the bedroom.

- Drink six to eight glasses (two quarts) of water a day.

- Breathe through your nose rather than through your mouth.

- Avoid antihistamines.

Home Treatment

- Follow the prevention guidelines.

Sjogren's Syndrome

Sjogren's (show-gruns) syndrome often accompanies rheumatoid arthritis. It causes dry mouth, itchy burning eyes, and vaginal dryness in women. In fact, 90 percent of all people with this disorder are postmenopausal women.

You cannot prevent or cure this syndrome, but you can help ease symptoms.

- For dry mouth, see the home treatment guidelines listed above.

- For dry eyes, see page 148.

- For vaginal dryness, see page 210.

- Practice good dental care. Lack of saliva increases your risk of tooth decay, so regular brushing and flossing are very important.

- Suck on sugarless candies or chew sugarless gum to increase salivation.

- Avoid caffeinated beverages, tobacco, and alcohol, all of which increase dryness in the mouth.

Taste Changes

As you age, you lose some of your sense of taste. Some of this taste loss may be linked to a decline in the sense of smell. However, there's no need to put up with poor taste! There are many preventable and reversible causes for taste loss:

- Viral infection

- Smoking

- Not thoroughly brushing both teeth and tongue

- Gum disease

- Dry mouth

- Medications--if you notice a marked decrease in taste when you are on any medication, report it to your doctor.

- Try saliva substitutes, such as Xerolube, which are available over-the-counter.

When to Call a Health Professional

- If dry mouth is causing difficulty in swallowing food.

- If dry mouth is accompanied by persistent sore throat.

- If dry mouth causes denture discomfort.

- If dry mouth is linked to medications that you are taking.

Laryngitis/ Hoarseness

Laryngitis is a viral or bacterial infection of the voice box (larynx). The most common cause is a cold, but it can also be produced by allergy. Symptoms of laryngitis are loss of voice, an urge to clear your throat, fever, tiredness, pain in the throat, and coughing. Hoarseness can be caused by yelling or cigarette smoke and displays symptoms similar to laryngitis.

Prevention

- If you have a respiratory infection, take time to treat it so that the infection won't spread to your voice box. See the home treatment guidelines on page 68.

Laryngitis - continued

- To prevent hoarseness, stop shouting as soon as you feel minor pain. Give your vocal cords a rest.

Home Treatment

- If hoarseness is caused by a cold, treat the cold. See page 68.

- Rest your voice by not shouting and by talking as little as possible.

- Stop smoking and avoid other people's smoke.

- Humidify the air.

- Drink lots of liquids.

Voice Changes

Some changes in the voice are normal as we age. Women may experience a lowering in pitch, while men's voices may get higher. Some people's voices may get hoarser or less clear.

There are other stresses on the voice: smoking, stroke, Parkinson's disease, vocal abuse (yelling, screaming, cheering), and a low level of thyroid hormone. Leading an inactive life also affects the voice. Keep physically and mentally active to help keep your voice strong.

- To soothe the throat, gargle with warm salt water (one teaspoon in eight ounces of water) or drink honey in hot water, lemon juice, or weak tea.

- Healing will take place within five to ten days. Medication will do little to speed recovery.

When to Call a Health Professional

- If you suspect a bacterial infection. See page 62.

- If hoarseness persists for one month.

Sore Throat/ Strep Throat

Often a mild sore throat is due to low humidity, smoking, air pollution, and, perhaps, yelling. People who have allergies or stuffy noses may breathe through their mouth while sleeping, causing a mild sore throat.

If you cannot determine the cause of a sore throat, or if you have been exposed to strep throat infections, you should get a throat culture.

Strep is a serious infection that must be diagnosed and treated by a health professional. It is usually, but not always, accompanied by a low (99°) or moderately high fever (103°), bright red throat, pus or white spots on the tonsils or throat, swollen neck glands, and severe pain.

Prevention

- Humidify your home, especially the bedroom.

- Identify and avoid irritants that cause sore throat (smoke, fumes, etc.).

- Don't smoke.

- Avoid contact with people who have strep throat.

Home Treatment

- Humidify the home, especially the bedroom.

- Gargle with warm salt water (one teaspoon in eight ounces of water). The salt reduces swelling.

- Some over-the-counter lozenges have a local anesthetic to deaden pain. Dyclonine hydrochloride (Sucrets Maximum Strength) and benzocaine (Spec-T and Tyrobenz) are considered safe and effective. Regular cough drops or hard candy may also soothe irritated tissue.

- If postnasal drip is present, gargle frequently to prevent chest colds and more throat irritation.

- Drink more fluids (at least two quarts a day) to soothe a sore throat. Honey and lemon or weak tea may help.

- Stop smoking.

When to Call a Health Professional

- If you cannot trace the cause of the sore throat.

- If someone in the family has recently had strep throat.

- If you have a history of frequent strep throats.

- If sore throat is accompanied by a fever higher than 99°.

- If a mild sore throat lasts longer than two weeks (becomes chronic).

- If the throat is very bright red, or has white spots or pus on it.

- Strep throat requires professional care and antibiotic treatment. Continue taking the antibiotic for the length of time prescribed (usually ten days). Do not stop even if you feel completely recovered. The full dose of antibiotic is needed to kill the bacteria and to prevent a quick recurrence of the infection.

TMJ Syndrome

The olive-sized joint that connects your jaw bone to your skull is called the temporomandibular joint (TMJ). TMJ syndrome is a set of symptoms that relate to damage, wear and tear, or unusual stress to the joint. The symptoms can include:

TMJ Syndrome - continued

- Joint pain at and around the joint

- Joint noises such as clicking, popping, or snapping

- Limited ability to "open wide"

- Muscle pain and spasms where the jaw muscles attach to the bone

- Headache, neck and shoulder pain, ear pain, eye pain, and difficulty swallowing

The cause of TMJ syndrome is difficult to determine. The most likely causes are:

- Direct trauma, such as a direct hit on the jaw

- Indirect trauma, such as whiplash

- Forceful stretching during dental work

- Chronic tooth grinding, clenching, or gum chewing

- Arthritis in the joint

- Chronic muscle tension due to stress, anxiety, depression, or poor posture. (This usually affects the jaw muscles more than the joint.)

- Teeth that do not meet when you bite

Conservative professional treatment for TMJ may involve a combination of the use of a plastic mouth plate (splint), physical therapy, and anti-inflammatory medications. Tooth filing, dental restorations, crowns or dentures may be needed later.

Surgery is needed for only a small percentage of TMJ problems. When needed, TMJ surgery is usually done by an oral surgeon. Before agreeing to surgery, talk with your physician and consider asking for a second opinion from a physician or dentist who has special training in TMJ problems. If surgery is needed, ask about arthroscopic surgery, which can be done on an outpatient basis.

Prevention

- Regularly practice progressive muscle relaxation, particularly before going to sleep. See page 302.

- Stop chewing gum or tough foods at the first sign that your jaw muscles are tiring.

- Good dentistry will allow your teeth to meet evenly when you bite down.

- Maintain good posture with your ear, shoulder, and hip in a straight line. See page 34.

Home Treatment

- Review and practice the tips for prevention.

- Avoid chewing gum.

- Avoid hard or chewy foods.

- Avoid opening your mouth too widely.

- Avoid cradling a telephone receiver between your shoulder and jaw.

- Rest your jaw, keeping your teeth apart and your lips closed. (Keep your tongue on the roof of your mouth, not between your teeth.)

- Put an ice pack on the joint for eight minutes, three times a day. Gently open and close your mouth while the ice pack is on. If the jaw muscle is swollen, increase to six times a day.

- Use aspirin or ibuprofen to reduce swelling and pain.

- If there is no swelling, use moist heat on the jaw muscle three times a day. Gently open and close your mouth while the heat is on. Alternate with the cold pack treatments.

- If you are under severe psychological stress or suffer from anxiety or depression, see Chapter 18, Mental Self-Care.

When to Call a Health Professional

Because there are over 50 different TMJ diagnoses, a dentist or physician with special training in TMJ may be needed to distinguish between a problem that can be resolved with home treatment and one that requires professional treatment. After the diagnosis, most problems can be solved with home treatment. Call your health professional:

- If pain is severe.

- If TMJ symptoms occur after direct or indirect trauma.

- If clicking or cracking sounds in your jaw continue without improvement for over two weeks.

- If any jaw dysfunction or pain continues without improvement for over two weeks.

- If other mild TMJ symptoms do not improve after four weeks of home treatment.

- After a diagnosis has ruled out "non-reducing disc displacement," ask your dentist/doctor to instruct you in exercises to restore a full range of motion to your jaw.

They aren't making mirrors like they used to.
Tallulah Bankhead

13

Skin, Hair, and Nails

The dry, rough, wrinkled skin of many older people is partly a result of the aging process. However, the degree of dryness, roughness, and wrinkling is due more to exposure to the sun than to age.

As a person ages, four changes in the skin are common:

- The outer layer of skin cells thins.

- The elasticity to hold skin tight decreases.

- The production of the protective oils that prevent dryness declines.

- The healing process for cuts and bruises slows down.

These changes are more pronounced and come earlier in people who have had lots of exposure to the sun during their lives.

The good news is that your skin usually outlasts your other vital organs. Except for skin cancers that are not caught early, death from skin problems is rare. No matter what skin, hair, and nail problems you have now, good self-care can help you to save your skin.

Age Spots

Age spots are changes in skin color caused by long-term exposure to sunlight. People used to think that the yellow, red, tan, or brown spots were a sign of liver ailments, hence the name liver spots. The spots cause no problems and have nothing to do with the liver. However, if the spots change in color, size, or shape, take the same precautions you would for any other skin changes. See page 195.

Blisters

Blisters are usually the result of persistent or repeated rubbing against the skin. Some illnesses, like shingles, cause blister-like rashes (see page 192). Burns can also blister the skin (see page 184).

Prevention

- Avoid shoes that are too tight or that rub on your toes or heels.

- Wear gloves to protect your hands when doing heavy chores.

- Wear sunscreen whenever you are outside to prevent blisters from sunburn.

Home Treatment

- If a blister is small and closed, it is best to leave it alone. Protect it from further rubbing with a loose bandage, and avoid the activity or shoes that caused it.

- If a blister is larger than one inch across, it is usually best to drain it. The following is a safe method:

  - Sterilize a needle by holding it in a flame from a match or lighter.

  - Gently puncture the blister at the edge.

  - Press the fluid in the blister toward the hole you have made to drain it.

- To treat a blister that has torn open, or one that you have opened to drain:

  - Wash the area with soap and water.

  - Do not remove the flap of skin that covered the blister unless it is very dirty or torn. Gently smooth it flat over the tender skin underneath.

  - Apply an antibacterial cream and a sterile bandage. Do not use alcohol or iodine. They will delay healing.

  - Remove the bandage at night to let the area dry.

  - Change the bandage once a day to reduce the chance of infection.

When to Call A Health Professional

- If blisters recur often and you do not know the cause.

- If signs of infection appear: redness, swelling, pain, or red streaks that extend away from the blister.

- If you have diabetes or peripheral vascular disease.

Boils

A boil is a red, swollen, painful bump under the skin, similar to an overgrown pimple. Boils occur most often in areas where there is hair and chafing. The neck, armpits, genitals, breasts, face, and buttocks are common boil sites.

Boils are often caused by an infected hair follicle. Bacteria from the infection will form an abscess or pocket of pus. The abscess can become as large as a ping-pong ball and be extremely painful.

Prevention

- Wash boil-prone areas often with soapy water. Dry thoroughly.

- Avoid clothing that is too tight or binding.

Home Treatment

- Do not squeeze, scratch, drain, or lance the boil. Squeezing can push the infection deeper into the skin. Scratching can spread the bacteria and form new boils.

- Use moist heat often. Keep hot, wet washcloths on the boil for 15 minutes at a time. The heat and moisture can help bring the boil to a head. Do this as soon as you notice the boil.

- Wash yourself well to prevent the boils from spreading.

When to Call a Health Professional

Your doctor can surgically drain the boil. The infection can be treated with antibiotics. Call the doctor if:

- The pain stops you from normal activities.

- You have a fever of 101° or higher.

- The boil is on your face or near your spine.

- The boil is not improving after two to three days of moist heat treatment.

- Any red streaking appears on the skin near the infected area.

- Any other lumps, particularly painful ones, develop near the infected area.

- You have diabetes.

Bruises

Aging and sun damage over the years weaken the tiny veins in the skin. The weakened veins are easily broken. This causes you to develop bruises more easily as you age. The bruises also take longer to heal than when you were younger.

The black and blue color of bruises is caused when blood cells seep from the veins into the skin tissue. Without a fresh supply of oxygen, the blood

Bruises - continued

turns dark blue. The blood will keep seeping until the tissue is saturated or the vein constricts.

Anticoagulant medications can react with aspirin and other drugs to cause easy bruising. Aspirin alone can also increase bruising in some people.

Home Treatment

- Apply ice or cold packs for 20 minute intervals during the first 48 hours after an injury to help the veins constrict. This will also reduce pain and swelling. The quicker you get a cold pack on the injury, the less bruising you will have.

- Elevate the bruised area. Blood will flow away from the injury.

- Rest the bruised area to allow the blood vessels to heal.

- After 48 hours, apply heat with warm towels, a hot water bottle, or a heating pad. This will increase circulation in the area to speed healing.

- Review all prescription and non-prescription drugs for possible drug interaction. Call your pharmacist or doctor to ask about drug interactions or side effects of medication.

When to Call a Health Professional

- If you suspect a drug interaction or if the following signs of infection develop:

  o Increasingly severe pain

  o Fever over 101°

  o Marked swelling and surrounding redness

- If you suddenly begin to bruise very easily.

- If you have unexplained recurrent or multiple bruises.

Burns

Burns are classified as first-, second-, or third-degree depending on their depth, not on the amount of pain nor the extent of the burn. A first-degree burn involves just the outer surface of the skin. The skin is dry, painful, and sensitive to touch. A mild sunburn is an example.

A second-degree burn involves the tissue beneath the skin in addition to the outer skin. The skin becomes swollen, puffy, weepy, or blistered.

A third-degree burn involves the outer skin, tissue beneath the skin, and any underlying tissue or organs. The skin is dry, pale white or charred black, swollen, and sometimes broken open. Nerves are destroyed or damaged, so there may be little pain except on the outer edges where there is a second-degree burn.

Prevention

Virtually all burns are preventable. Here is what you can do to prevent fires and burns in your home:

- Quit smoking--especially in bed.

- Replace worn electrical cords.

- Don't overload electrical outlets.

- Have wood stove or fireplace chimneys cleaned at least once a year. Keep newspapers away from fireplaces and stoves.

- Use space heaters with caution. Keep them clear of curtains, paper, etc. Avoid placing them in areas where they could be tipped over.

- Keep a fire extinguisher near the kitchen. Have it inspected yearly.

- Install smoke alarms in kitchen and sleeping areas. Replace batteries regularly.

- Set your water heater at 120° or lower to avoid burns.

- Use caution when using heating pads and electric blankets. Do not fall asleep with a heating pad on your skin.

- See additional fire prevention tips on page 23.

Home Treatment

- For home treatment of sunburn, see page 194.

- Run cold tap water over the burn immediately. Ice or cold water is the best immediate treatment for minor burns. The cold lowers the skin temperature and lessens the severity of the burn. Switch to ice when you can.

- Prepare for swelling. Remove rings from burned hands.

- Do not put any salves, butter, grease, oils, or lubricants on a burn. They increase the risk of infection and don't help to heal the burn.

- The juice from a broken aloe leaf can soothe minor burns.

- Do not cover the burn unless it rubs against clothing. If it rubs, it is better to cover the wound than to break open the blisters. To cover a burn, remove any burned clothing. Wash the burned area and cover it with a single layer of gauze. Tape the edges of the gauze well away from the burned area. Do not encircle a hand, arm or leg with tape. Swelling may later make the tape too tight. This dressing needs to be changed the following day and then every two days.

Burns - continued

- A third-degree burn needs immediate medical treatment. Do not apply any salves or medication since these will have to be removed later for treatment and their removal may cause further harm. The burned person should lie down to reduce the risk of shock.

When to Call a Health Professional

- If a second-degree burn involves the face, hands, feet, genitals, or a joint.

- If the burn encircles an arm or leg or covers more than one-quarter of the body part involved.

- If the pain lasts longer than 48 hours.

- If in doubt as to extent of burn, or in doubt if it is a second- or third-degree burn.

- For all third-degree burns.

- If an infection starts developing. Signs of infection are:

  o Fever of 101° or higher

  o Increase in pain, redness, and swelling

  o Drainage of pus

Dry Skin/Itching

As you age, your skin produces less of the natural oils that help retain its moisture. By age 70, a majority of people experience dryness and itchiness on their lower legs, forearms, hands, and scalp. Without good home care, the skin can become red, cracked, and prone to irritations and infections.

Prevention

- Avoid overexposure to the sun. See page 194.

- Humidify your home, particularly the bedroom.

- Drink at least two quarts of water every day.

- Avoid vigorous, hot water washing because it removes all of the skin's natural oils. Warm or cool water washing is more gentle on the skin.

- Avoid detergents and deodorant soaps.

- Avoid extensive use of perfumes and perfumed products.

Home Treatment

- Follow the prevention guidelines above.

- Avoid scratching. It damages the skin.

- Use moisturizing creams or lotions to restore lost oils to the skin. Lubriderm and Keri Lotion are good.

- Bathe every other day instead of every day. Use little or no soap on dry skin areas. Use cool or warm bath water. Pat yourself dry. Do not rub your skin vigorously with either washcloths or towels. Apply a moisturizer while your skin is still damp. Petroleum jelly (Vaseline) is an inexpensive and effective moisturizer.

- For very dry hands, wash with lotion instead of soap. Wipe off the excess with a soft towel.

- For home treatment of rashes, see page 191.

When to Call a Health Professional

- If you itch all over your body without obvious cause or rash.

- If itching is so bad that you cannot sleep and home treatment methods are not helping.

- If the skin is badly broken due to scratching.

Relief From Itching

- Keep the area cool and wet. Try a compress soaked in water or Burrow's solution, which is available at the drugstore.

- Aspirin can help relieve itching.

- Alpha-Keri and Syntex are bath oils that are excellent for dry, itching skin. Use them very sparingly.

- An oatmeal bath may help relieve itching. Wrap a cup of oatmeal in a cotton cloth and boil as you would to cook it. Use this as a sponge and bathe in tepid water without soap.

- Try over-the-counter hydrocortisone for local areas of itching.

- If itching is very severe, your doctor may prescribe a stronger cream.

- Try an over-the-counter antihistamine such as Chlor-Trimeton or Benadryl. See precautions about antihistamines on page 333.

Foot Problems

There is a long list of foot problems that cause pain or concern. Here are a few:

- Athlete's foot: a fungal infection that causes cracks and peeling between the toes.

- Bunions: bony knobs that protrude from the inner sides of the balls of the feet, just below the big toe. See page 43.

- Calluses and corns: hard, thickened skin on parts of the foot exposed to friction.

- Hammer toe: a permanent downward bending of the middle joint of a toe. See page 43.

- Plantar wart: a wart on the heel or ball of your foot. It may look like a callus with tiny pin holes or spots in the center.

- Also see Gout on page 46.

Most of these problems can be prevented with proper foot care.

Prevention

- Wear shoes that have plenty of room for your foot. Buy comfortable shoes that make your feet feel good. Because your feet swell during the day, try on and buy your shoes in the late afternoon. Running shoes, walking shoes, or lightweight hiking boots may be best. Avoid shoes with pointed toes or high heels. Women with wide feet may be able to find better-fitting shoes in the men's department.

- Keep your feet clean and dry. If your feet sweat a lot, use cornstarch powder between your toes, wear cotton socks, and change them often.

- Massage your feet. It feels great and relieves tension.

Home Treatment

Note special foot care for people with diabetes on page 122.

- Follow prevention guidelines above.

- For athlete's foot:

  ○ Wear cotton socks to absorb perspiration.

  ○ Change your socks twice a day.

  ○ Alternate your pairs of shoes from day to day.

  ○ Use antifungal powders, sprays, or creams like Tinactin or Desenex.

- For bunions (also see page 43):

  ○ Exercise foot muscles to improve circulation.

  ○ Try arch supports.

  ○ Wear shoes with plenty of room for the toes.

- For calluses and corns:

  o Soak your feet in warm water.

  o Rub the area with an emery board or pumice stone.

  o Apply a 40 percent salicylic acid plaster overnight. Repeat as needed.

- For hammer toe (also see page 43):

  o Wear roomy shoes.

  o Massage and exercise the foot.

  o Wear small pads on top of the middle joint to relieve shoe pressure.

  o If the toe is flexible, consider toe splints to hold the toe flat.

- For plantar warts (also see page 197):

  o Use doughnut-shaped foam rubber pads to relieve pressure when you walk.

  o Use salicylic acid plasters.

  o Avoid direct contact between the wart and other body parts.

When to Call a Health Professional

- If you have diabetes or peripheral vascular disease and develop foot problems. Also see page 122.

- If signs of infection develop (redness, pus, swelling, pain).

- If the condition is very painful or it worsens after home treatment.

- If the condition does not improve after two to three weeks of home treatment.

Hair Changes

As your skin ages and hormones change, your hair may also undergo changes. Men tend to lose hair. After menopause, women tend to grow more facial and body hair. Both men and women tend to lose hair color. All of these changes are normal and none pose medical problems. The only risk that baldness brings is that of scalp sunburn, so use sunscreen on your head, or wear a hat. For more information on baldness, see page 217.

Bald spots, however, should be distinguished from baldness. Bald spots for men or for women may be caused by repeated stress to the hair such as tight braids or habitual hair pulling. Bald spots that occur on a normal scalp may sometimes indicate a more serious problem.

Some medications, vitamins, and illnesses may cause hair to break near the roots, change texture, or come out easily. Consult a physician if this occurs.

Hair Changes - continued

When to Call a Health Professional

- Call your doctor if you do not know the cause of any bald spot.

Nail Problems

With good care, most fingernails and toenails will stay healthy and trouble-free for a lifetime. However, after years of poor care or abuse from ill-fitting shoes, toenails can get into trouble.

Thickened and curved nails can be caused by repeated bruising, inflammation, infection, or disease. The nail is often discolored and may be painful.

Ingrown toenail is caused when an improperly trimmed toenail cuts into the skin at the edge of the nail. Because the cut can easily become infected, prompt care is needed.

Prevention

- Cut toenails straight across so that edges cannot cut into skin.

- Wear roomy shoes.

- Wash feet and change socks often.

Home Treatment

- For ingrown toenails:

  ○ Soak your foot in warm water.

  ○ Wedge a small piece of wet tissue under the corner of the nail to help it grow out straight.

  ○ Trim the offending nail.

When to Call a Health Professional

- If signs of infection develop (redness, pus, swelling, pain).

- If yellow-brown discoloration, nail destruction, or other signs of fungal infection develop.

- If you also have diabetes or circulatory problems.

Caregiver Tips on Nail Care

People with poor eyesight, stiffness, or tremor may have difficulty providing proper nail care for themselves. Present them with the gift of a foot bath, foot massage, and toenail and fingernail trim every few weeks. Use care when trimming toenails and fingernails for a person who has diabetes or peripheral vascular disease.

Rashes

A rash (dermatitis) is any irritation or inflammation of the skin. Rashes can be caused by illness, allergy, heat, or emotional stress. When you first get a rash, ask yourself the following questions to help determine its cause:

- Did the rash follow contact with anything new that could have irritated your skin: poison ivy, detergents, shampoos, perfumes, lotions, etc.?

- Have you eaten anything that you may be allergic to?

- Are you taking any new medications, either prescription or over-the-counter?

- Have you been unusually stressed or upset recently?

- Is there a fever with the rash?

- Is there joint pain with the rash?

- Is the rash spreading?

- Does the rash itch?

Seborrheic Dermatitis

Older adults are particularly prone to outbreaks of seborrheic dermatitis. Small reddish-yellow scaly patches develop in skin areas that are particularly oily: the scalp, forehead, sides of the nose, eyelids, behind the ears, and in the center of the chest.

This common problem is caused by overactive oil glands in the skin. Emotional stress, physical exertion, and certain medications can trigger flare-ups. It responds well to home treatment with dandruff shampoos and mild steroid creams.

Intertrigo (Chafing)

Intertrigo is a chafing rash that occurs between body skin folds. Common sites are the armpit, groin, inner thighs, anal region, and under the breasts. Moisture, warmth, and friction combine to cause chafing of the skin.

Weight loss and home treatment can clear up the problem before bacterial or fungal infections develop.

Home Treatment

- Watch for early signs of rashes. Fast treatment can usually resolve the problem quickly, before it spreads.

- Wash affected areas with water. Soap can be irritating. Pat dry thoroughly.

- Apply cold, wet washcloths to reduce itching. Repeat frequently. For relief of itching, see page 187.

- Leave the rash exposed to the air. Cornstarch or baby powder can be helpful to keep it dry. Avoid lotions and ointments until the rash heals. Hydrocortisone cream can provide temporary relief of itching. Ask your pharmacist.

- Lose weight to reduce skin folds. See page 295.

Rashes - continued

When to Call a Health Professional

- If signs of infection appear (redness, pus, swelling, pain).

- If a fever of 101° or higher develops.

- If you suspect the rash is the result of a medication reaction.

- If there is severe pain in a joint.

Shingles

Some people who had chicken pox as children may develop shingles later in life. Shingles (herpes zoster) is caused by the reactivation of the chicken pox virus in the body. The virus usually affects one of the large nerves that spread outward from the spine, causing pain and a rash in a band around one side of the chest, abdomen, or face.

The symptoms of shingles develop in a pattern. First, there will be a tingling, burning, throbbing, or stabbing pain in the affected nerve. If the virus is affecting a nerve in the chest wall, the pain may mimic that of a heart attack.

A rash, which develops into blisters, will appear two to three days after the pain begins. The blisters will dry up in a few days and will drop off in two to three weeks.

About half of people over 60 who get shingles experience lingering pain (post-herpetic neuralgia) in the affected nerve for months or years.

No one is sure what causes the chicken pox virus to become active again. Shingles may be more likely to develop when medications or illness have weakened a person's immune system.

Prevention

- If you have never had chicken pox, avoid exposure to people with shingles or chicken pox.

- A vaccine to prevent shingles has passed preliminary tests and may become available in the future.

Home Treatment

- Keep the blisters clean and dry to prevent infection.

- Reduce the pain from your clothing rubbing against the blisters by taping cotton gauze over the blistered area.

- See page 187 for relief from itching.

- Use aspirin or acetaminophen to control minor pain.

- Avoid contact with children, pregnant women, and adults who have never had chicken pox until the blisters have completely dried.

When to Call a Health Professional

- Call immediately if the chest pain comes with any other symptoms of heart attack: shortness of breath, dizziness, nausea, sweating, weakness. See page 84.

- If you suspect shingles, call your doctor to discuss drugs that can limit the pain and rash.

- If shingles appear in or near the eye.

- If facial pain develops, get medical treatment promptly to limit damage to your eyes.

Skin Growths

Non-Cancerous Growths
Most bumps and lumps that occur as we age are harmless growths, spots, or tabs that remain stable once they have appeared. These include:

- Seborrheic keratoses: circular, brown/black, waxy, wart-like, low-profile growths on face, neck, and trunk. Their color fades if they are protected from sunlight.

- Cherry angiomas (ruby spots): small, reddish-purple spots most often found on the trunk and upper legs, but also on face, neck, scalp and arms. These harmless clusters of dilated capillaries are increasingly common after age 40. They will bleed profusely if punctured.

- Skin tags: fleshy, tag-like growths of skin on the face, neck, chest, and arms.

- Sebaceous gland growths: yellowish bumps over the forehead and face.

Pre-Cancerous Growths/Patches
Solar or actinic keratoses is the name given to small red patches caused by long-term exposure to sunlight. These patches have a few visible blood vessels and a yellow-brown surface. They are often pre-cancerous. If protected from the sun, the patches may grow smaller and disappear. If sun exposure continues, they may eventually change into skin cancers in five to fifteen years.

Prevention and Home Treatment

- Always protect these patches and the rest of your skin with sunscreens that have a sun protective factor (SPF) of 15 or greater.

When to Call a Health Professional

- If a pigmented mark or elevation appears or changes size, shape, texture, or color.

- If a sore persists for four to six weeks without healing.

- If signs of skin cancer develop. See next page.

Skin Cancer

Skin cancer is the most common of all cancers. Fortunately, it is also the easiest to cure.

Most skin cancer is caused by earlier sun damage to the skin. Ninety percent of skin problems occur on the face, neck, and arms, where sun exposure is greatest.

Light-skinned, blue-eyed people are more likely to develop skin cancer. Dark-skinned people have less risk.

Skin cancer is generally slow-growing, easy to recognize, and easy to treat by simple removal in a doctor's office. A small percentage of skin cancers are much more serious.

Basal cell cancer

This is the most common type of skin cancer. It affects the cells beneath the skin. The tumors vary widely in appearance. Look for pinkish, solid nodules, red spots, white areas like scar tissue, or skin ulcers that don't heal. They are rarely fatal, but can cause cosmetic problems. They are slow-growing and easily removed.

Squamous cell cancer

This type of cancer is less frequent but more hazardous because it can spread to other organs. These growths generally cause more of a raised or lumpy looking growth. They tend to bleed more easily. Treatment is much more urgent.

Avoiding Sunburn

Sunburn is completely preventable. If you are going to be in the sun for more than 15 minutes, take the following precautions.

- Use a sunscreen with a sun protective factor (SPF) of at least 15.

- Apply the sunscreen 15 minutes before exposure. Reapply every two hours.

- If you are allergic to PABA, the active ingredient in most sunscreens, use non-PABA alternatives. Ask your pharmacist.

- Wear a broad-brimmed hat that will shade your face.

- Wear light-colored, loose-fitting, long-sleeved clothes.

- Drink lots of water. Sweating helps to cool the skin and lessen damage.

Please note: Some sunshine on the skin is needed to produce vitamin D. Vitamin D and calcium are needed to strengthen bones against osteoporosis.

Since sunscreens block vitamin D production, you must balance your need to protect your skin with your need to protect your bones. One solution is to drink lots of vitamin D-fortified milk. Another is to take a low-dosage vitamin D supplement. (No more than 1000 IU per day.)

These skin cancers are easily identified and can be removed in a physician's office.

Skin cancers of the non-melanoma type tend to develop in sun-exposed areas. They differ from non-cancerous growths in several important ways:

- Skin cancers tend to bleed more. They are often open sores.

- Skin cancers usually feel firm, not fleshy, to the touch.

- Skin cancers tend to keep growing, even if the growth is slow.

Malignant melanomas (cancerous moles)

Most moles are harmless. However, malignant melanomas can be fatal if not promptly treated. They grow rapidly and often spread (metastasize). Without prompt treatment, melanomas can be fatal. They account for about 5,000 deaths a year in the U.S.

Make an immediate appointment with your doctor if a mole or other pigmented area shows any of the following:

- Asymmetrical shape: One half does not match the other half.

- Border irregularity: The edges are ragged, notched, or blurred.

- Color: The color is not uniform. Shades of tan, brown, and black are present. Red, white, and blue may add to the mottled appearance.

- Diameter: Larger than a pencil eraser. Harmless moles are usually smaller.

- Scaliness, oozing, bleeding, or the spread of pigment into surrounding skin.

- Appearance of a bump or nodule on the mole.

- Itching, tenderness, or pain.

Asymmetrical Shape

Border Irregular

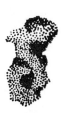

Color Varied

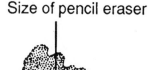

Size of pencil eraser

Mole

Diameter larger than a pencil eraser

Mole Changes to Watch For

Skin Cancer - continued

Prevention

Most skin cancers can be prevented by avoiding heavy exposure to the sun. Unfortunately, sun damage from earlier years can be the cause of skin cancer later in life.

Home Treatment

- Avoid further sun damage to the skin. See Avoiding Sunburn on page 194.

- Examine your skin with the help of another person or a mirror, once a month. Look for unusual moles, spots, or bumps. Be especially attentive to areas of your skin that received a lot of sun exposure earlier in your life: hands, arms, chest and neck (including the back of the neck), face, ears, etc. Note any changes and report to your doctor.

When to Call a Health Professional

If you detect any of the signs of skin cancer and malignant melanomas, call your doctor.

Warts

Warts are skin growths that are caused by a virus. They can appear anywhere on the body. Warts are not dangerous, but can be very bothersome.

Little is known about warts. Most are only slightly contagious. They can spread to other areas on the same person but rarely to others. Genital and anal warts are exceptions; they are sexually transmitted and are a risk factor in cancer of the cervix. See page 214.

Because warts seem to come and go for little reason, it's possible that they are sensitive to slight changes in the immune system. In some cases, one can "think" them away.

When necessary, your health professional can remove warts by freezing them, by electrolysis, by cutting them off, or with chemicals. Unfortunately, they often come back or leave a scar.

Home Treatment

- Warts appear and disappear spontaneously. They can last a week, a month, or even years. To get rid of your warts, it helps to believe in the treatment. If something works for you, stick with it.

- If the wart bleeds a little, cover it with a bandage and apply light pressure to stop the bleeding.

- If the wart is in the way, use a pumice stone or a mild ointment containing 5% salicylic acid. These are over-the-counter products. Ask your pharmacist for help.

- Plantar warts appear on the feet and can be painful. You can buy doughnut-shaped foam rubber pads that alleviate the pressure on the wart when you walk. Use pads if they relieve pain and the wart doesn't increase in size. Otherwise, see your health professional.

- Try the least expensive method of treating warts that you can think of. You may save a trip to your health professional.

- Don't attempt to cut or burn off a wart yourself.

When to Call a Health Professional

- If the wart has been irritated or knocked off. It could become infected.

- If a plantar wart is painful when you walk, and foam pads do not help.

- If you have warts in the anal or genital area. See page 232.

- If the wart causes continued discomfort.

- If a wart develops on the face and is of cosmetic concern.

Flowers wilt and candy's sweet,
but thermal socks will warm your feet.
Unknown

14

Temperature Control Problems

Everyone has heard that normal body temperature is 98.6°F. That is the normal line on most oral thermometers. However, there is more to the story. "Normal" is not the same for everyone. Your own normal temperature may vary from 97.6° to 99.6°. You may also find that your normal temperature is about a degree lower in the early morning than it is in the evening. Vigorous exercise will often increase body temperature for several hours.

The hypothalamus is the part of the brain that controls the body's temperature. When your body gets too hot, the hypothalamus works to increase the blood flow to the skin to help you cool off. Sweat glands also help reduce body heat through evaporation.

When you are too cold, the hypothalamus reduces the blood flow to the skin and shuts down the sweat glands. It also triggers goose bumps, which make your hair stand up for better insulation.

This chapter covers the basics of temperature control problems, from cold hands and feet to fevers. You will also find specific guidelines to follow when prolonged exposure to heat or cold causes heat stroke or hypothermia.

Cold Hands and Feet

Many older adults suffer from cold hands and feet. Exposure to even mildly cold temperatures causes the blood vessels in their fingers and toes to constrict. In some people, the hands and feet may appear white. A condition called Raynaud's syndrome is often the cause. It is thought to be a complication of any of several underlying illnesses that inhibit circulation. Sometimes, no cause can be found.

Cold Hands/Feet - continued

Prevention

- Avoid or cut back on caffeinated coffee, tea, and colas.

- Quit smoking.

- Avoid tranquilizers, sleeping pills, antidepressants, and alcohol.

- Practice progressive muscle relaxation. See page 302.

- Get regular exercise.

Home Treatment

- Follow the prevention guidelines.

- Whirl your arms around like a windmill to bring more blood into the fingers.

- Wear warm socks and gloves in cool weather. Cover your head, too. Thirty percent of your body heat escapes through your head.

- Soak hands and feet in warm water for five minutes before bedtime.

When to Call a Health Professional

- If pain accompanies feelings of coldness.

- If hands or feet are cold and white with no feeling.

- If skin ulcers or open sores are present.

- If only one hand or foot is cold.

Fever

The increased body temperature that comes with a fever helps the body to fight infection. Generally, fever acts to help you recover from illness more quickly.

The degree of the fever is not always related to the severity of the infection. This is particularly true for older adults. As you age, your body may lose some of its ability to create a fever. An 80-year-old pneumonia patient with a fever of 100° may be just as sick as a 24-year-old pneumonia patient with a fever of 105°.

Many symptoms that normally accompany high fever can develop in older adults without the usual increase in body temperature. These symptoms include headache, dizziness, restlessness, confusion, delusions, and paranoia. If these symptoms do appear, serious infections could be present even though fever is not apparent. Subnormal temperatures (94°) may indicate infection or thyroid problems. Temperatures above or below what is normal for you can be an important clue to illness.

In older adults, a high fever can place an increased strain on the heart. For people with heart disease, a high fever can sometimes trigger heart failure. Fevers in older adults are

---

also more likely to cause delirium or disorientation than in younger people.

Four Levels of Fever

Mild Fever   (99° to 100°)
1 to 2 degrees above normal

Moderate Fever   (101° to 102°)
 3 to 4 degrees above normal

High Fever   (103° to 104°)
5 to 6 degrees above normal

Very High Fever   (105°+)
7 or more degrees above normal

Home Treatment

The treatment of fever in older adults depends on what other symptoms accompany it. A fever will cause an increase in blood flow and metabolism rates that may speed healing. A mild or moderate fever (up to 102°) with no other symptoms of distress may just need watching.

- Drink at least 10 glasses of water a day to replenish liquids lost because of the fever. (Consult your doctor before increasing fluids if you have congestive heart failure.)

- Eat light, easily digested foods such as clear soups.

- Retake and record the temperature every waking hour.

If a high fever or symptoms of a high fever develop (headaches, dizziness, confusion, delusions, etc.), it is important to reduce the fever. A high

fever may be reduced in one or more of the following ways:

- Use sponges or wet cloths with lukewarm (70°) water to cool the body by evaporation.

- Take two regular aspirin every four hours with lots of water. Stick to a regular four hour schedule to prevent the fever from going up. Acetaminophen (Tylenol) will also work fine, and causes less stomach irritation.

- High fevers need to be evaluated by a doctor. In the meantime:

  ○ To bring down a high fever (over 103°), apply cool washcloths or cold packs to neck, armpits, and groin.

  ○ If the temperature is very high (105° or higher), soak in a cool water bath until the temperature starts to come down.

  ○ If the temperature is 106° or higher, add ice to a cold water bath to bring the fever down faster. If cooling lowers the temperature below 102°, use care to avoid overcooling.

When to Call a Health Professional

- If an older person who is frail or in poor health has a fever that is 101° or higher. For generally healthy older adults, call a health professional:

Fever - continued

- o If a fever reaches 104°.

- o If a fever of unknown cause stays at 101° or higher for three full days.

- o If delirium or confusion comes with any fever.

- If you have fever and any of the following symptoms, see the referenced pages for additional guidelines:

  - o Shortness of breath and cough. See Pneumonia on page 73 and Bronchitis on page 62.

  - o Pain over your eyes or cheeks. See Sinusitis, page 74.

  - o Pain or burning when you urinate. See Urinary Tract Infection, page 115.

  - o Abdominal pain, nausea, and vomiting. See Food Poisoning/Stomach Flu, page 103.

- Call your doctor if a fever is associated with any disturbing or unexplained symptoms.

Heat Exhaustion/ Heat Stroke

Heat exhaustion occurs when your body cannot sweat enough to cool you off. Generally, it happens when you are working or exercising in hot weather. The symptoms of heat exhaustion include fatigue, dizziness, nausea, and weakness. The skin will be cool, clammy, and pale.

Prevention

- Avoid strenuous outdoor physical activity during the hottest part of the day.

- Wear light-colored, loose-fitting clothing to reflect the sun.

- Avoid sudden changes of temperature. Air out hot cars before getting into them.

- Drink 8 to 10 glasses of water per day.

- If you take diuretics, ask your physician about a lower dosage during hot weather.

Home Treatment

- Get out of the sun to a cool spot.

- Drink lots of water.

- If you are nauseated or dizzy, lie down awhile in a cool spot and then start taking water a little at a time.

- If the body temperature reaches 105°, immediate cooling is essential. Use cold, wet cloths all over the body. An ice water bath may be necessary.

- If cooling lowers the temperature to 102°, use care to avoid over-cooling.

When to Call a Health Professional

Heat exhaustion can sometimes lead to heat stroke, particularly in older adults. Heat stroke occurs when the body stops sweating, even though the body temperature continues to rise. If you find any of the following symptoms of heat stroke, work fast to lower the body temperature and seek immediate help:

- The skin is dry, even under the armpits.

- The body temperature reaches 104° and keeps rising.

- The person is delirious, disoriented, or unconscious.

- The skin is bright red.

Hypothermia

Hypothermia occurs when the body's core temperature drops below normal. It is caused when the body loses heat faster than heat can be produced by muscle contraction and shivering.

The symptoms of hypothermia include mental confusion, apathy, restlessness, shivering, and hallucinations. The person may or may not complain of being cold. The body temperature will drop below normal and continue to fall. The person will feel cold and his abdomen will be cold, pale, and waxy-looking. The heart rate slows and respiration becomes slow and irregular.

Hypothermia is an emergency. It can quickly lead to unconsciousness and death if the heat loss continues. It is a particular problem for older adults in cold climates. Air temperature, wind, and wetness all affect the rate at which heat leaves the body. Hypothermia can happen at temperatures of 45°, or even higher in wet and windy weather. Very frail and inactive people can become hypothermic indoors if they are not dressed warmly.

People who have heart disease or diabetes, or who are inactive due to arthritis, stroke, or other conditions are at increased risk of hypothermia. Certain medications, including those used to treat high blood pressure, antidepressents, narcotics, barbiturates, sleeping pills, and anxiety drugs also increase the risk of hypothermia.

Prevention

- Get up and move around regularly if you must be indoors during cold weather. If mobility is a problem, do chair exercises or other activities that will get your blood moving.

Hypothermia - continued

- Avoid alcoholic beverages, which increase heat loss and may also make you less likely to notice that you are becoming chilled.

- Eat regular, healthy meals. Your body needs calories to produce heat.

- Keep windows closed during cold weather. People over 65 should keep indoor temperature at least 65°.

- Avoid taking sleeping pills.

- Wear warm clothes to bed at night and use warm bedding.

- Dress warmly in layers and carry water-proof clothing when outside. Wool and some other materials remain warm even when wet. Cotton does not.

- Wear a warm hat and gloves.

- Eat well before going out on a cold day and carry food to increase your energy.

- Take shelter if you get wet or cold.

Home Treatment

The goal of home or "in-the-field" treatment is to stop additional heat loss and slowly rewarm the person.

- For mild cases, get the person out of the cold and wind, have them put on either dry or wool clothing, and ask them to drink warm fluids.

- For moderate cases, use your own body heat to warm the person by wrapping yourself and the victim in the same blanket or sleeping bag. Remove cold, wet clothes first.

- Do not attempt to give food or drink to an unconscious person.

- Do not provide alcoholic beverages.

- Rewarming the victim in warm water can cause shock or heart attack. However, in emergency situations where professional help is not available, and other home treatments are not working, you can use a warm water soak as a last resort.

When to Call a Health Professional

- If the person loses consciousness or at any time seems confused.

- If the body temperature does not return to normal after four hours of warming.

- If the person is frail.

*The most creative force in the world
is the menopausal woman with zest.*
Margaret Mead

15
Women's Health

Women have special health needs when it comes to self care. From puberty to menopause, women must cope with health care problems that are unique to them. This chapter covers health issues of special concern to older women and what you can do to manage them better.

Breast Health

After lung cancer, breast cancer is the second leading cause of cancer deaths in women. However, breast cancer is highly curable if it is detected early. There are three methods to use for early detection: breast self-exam, a doctor's physical exam, and a mammogram.

Breast Self-Exam

Most breast lumps are discovered by women themselves, often quite by accident. The breast self-exam is a simple technique to help you learn what is normal for you and to become aware of any changes.

Set up a regular time each month to examine your breasts. The first day of each month is an easy time to remember.

Most women's breast tissue has some lumpiness or thickening. This is common. When in doubt about a particular lump, check the other breast. If you find a similar lump in the same area on the other breast, both breasts are probably normal. Be on the lookout for a lump that feels much harder than the rest of the breast.

You can have any areas of concern or doubt checked out by your doctor. The important thing is to learn what is usual **for you** and to report changes to your doctor.

The breast self-exam takes place in three stages.

Breast Self-Exam - continued

Stage 1: In the bath or shower

Begin your breast exam in the shower or bath, when your hands are wet and soapy and can glide easily over the skin. Using the flat surfaces of your fingers (not your fingertips), gently move over every part of each breast and armpit. Check for unusual lumps or thickening.

Place your palms on your hips and press down firmly to flex your chest muscles. Again, look for dimpling or any skin changes.

Next, squeeze the nipple of each breast gently between thumb and index finger. Look for a discharge.

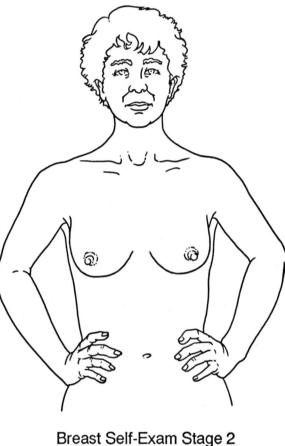

Breast Self-Exam Stage 2

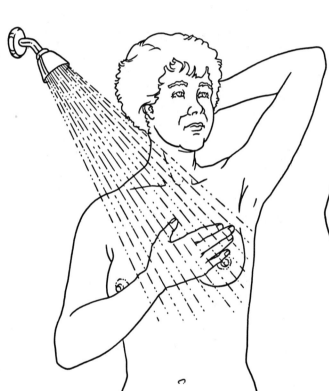

Breast Self-Exam Stage 1

Stage 2: In front of the mirror

Look at your breasts in a mirror. Few women have breasts that match exactly. Learn what is normal for you. Look for any dimpling or puckering of the skin, or any changes in the contour and shape of the breast.

Stage 3: Lying down

Place a pillow or folded towel under your left shoulder and position your left arm under your head. Use your right hand to examine your left breast. With fingers relaxed, move the flat surface of your fingers in a gentle, circular motion to examine the breast. Feel for lumps, thickening, or changes of any kind.

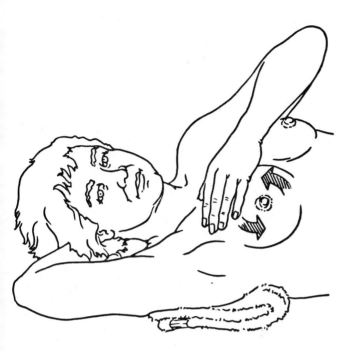

Breast Self-Exam Stage 3

To make sure you cover the whole area, imagine that your breast is a clock. Start on the outside of the breast at 12:00, move slowly to 1:00 and then around the clock back to 12:00. Then move one inch in toward the nipple and go around the "clock" again. Be sure to include the nipple, the breastbone, and the armpit in your exam.

Move the pillow or towel to the other shoulder and repeat this procedure for the other breast.

If you discover any unusual lumps, thickening, or changes of any kind, report them to your doctor. Remember, most lumps are not malignant, but you will need your doctor to make a diagnosis.

If you start a habit of examining your breasts monthly, you will learn what is normal for you and quickly recognize if something changes. The breast self-exam does take some practice. Ask your doctor for help in learning the technique.

Doctor's Physical Exam

The second component for early detection of breast problems is your doctor's physical exam. An annual breast exam is recommended.

Mammogram

Mammograms, which are breast x-rays, find tumors too small to be detected by a breast self-exam. Mammograms are recommended every one to two years for women between the ages of 50 and 75. Annual mammograms are advised for women receiving estrogen replacement therapy and women who are at higher risk for breast cancer. See page 216.

Regular screening could lead to a 30 percent drop in breast cancer deaths. However, less than a third of older women follow recommended guidelines for regular mammograms. Don't put it off. Your local hospital or American Cancer Society chapter can provide information on where to get a mammogram.

Breast Health Tips

- Get smart about early detection. If detected early, breast cancer can be cured 90 percent of the time.

  - Do the breast self-exam every month.

  - Have a doctor's physical exam every year.

  - Have a mammogram every one to two years, or yearly if you have one or more risk factors for breast cancer. See "Risk Factors for Women's Cancers" on page 216.

- Eat a low-fat diet. Cut down on fried foods and high-fat dairy products.

- Eat foods containing vitamins A and C (dark green and orange vegetables and fruits).

- Eat more cruciferous vegetables (broccoli, cabbage, kale).

Gynecological Health

Pelvic exams and Pap smears are vital components of women's health. The exams are important because they give you early signs of any abnormalities in your reproductive organs.

Regular pelvic exams are also important for women who have had a hysterectomy. Even if your uterus and ovaries have been removed, you are not immune to cancer of the cervix, vagina and vulva.

Periodically examine your entire genital area for any sores, warts, red swollen areas, or unusual vaginal discharge. A healthy vaginal discharge will be white to yellowish-white and smell slightly like vinegar. It can be either thick or thin and present in large or small amounts; every woman is different.

There should be no pain or straining on urination. If you experience pain or burning on urination, read about Urinary Tract Infections on page 115.

The Pelvic Exam

A pelvic exam given by a health care professional will consist of an external genital exam, a Pap test, and a manual exam, generally in that order.

The Pap test is the screening exam for cancer of the cervix. Pap smears detect 90 percent to 95 percent of cervical cancers, making this a reliable and important test. See Women's Cancers on page 213.

Schedule pelvic exams and Pap smears every two to three years. After age 65 you can stop the Pap smears **after** two consecutive normal tests. Continue with the rest of the pelvic exam. Women who have had a hysterectomy need regular Pap smears also, unless the cervix has been removed.

Menopause

Menopause occurs for most women between the ages of 45 and 55 (the average age is 51) when the production of the "female hormones," estrogen and progesterone, is greatly reduced. With these hormonal changes, you may experience irregular menstrual periods before they stop altogether. You may also experience hot flashes, vaginal dryness, and mood changes. Osteoporosis is also directly linked to the decrease in estrogen that comes with menopause. See page 50.

You are considered to have passed menopause after one year of no menstrual periods. Because women can expect to spend one-third of their lives after menopause, management of menopause-related problems is very important.

Irregular Periods may mean lighter or heavier than usual menstrual flows, shorter or longer intervals between flows, or spotting. Some women experience irregular periods for years in association with menopause. Others have regular periods until they suddenly stop. Every woman is unique and will experience menopause differently.

Hot Flashes are sudden periods of intense heat, sweating, and flushing. They are experienced by 75 percent to 80 percent of women going through menopause. They may occur as frequently as once an hour and last as long as three to four minutes. A hot flash usually begins in the chest and spreads out to the neck, face, and arms. Hot flashes usually cease within one or two years.

Another side effect of hot flashes is what they do to your sleep patterns. Hot flashes that occur during sleep can wake you up. Disrupted sleep patterns can lead to insomnia, fatigue, irritability, and poor concentration.

Vaginal Changes that occur with menopause include dryness and loss of elasticity, thinning of the vaginal walls, and shrinking of the labia, the outer lips of the vagina. Pain, irritation, and discharge resulting from these changes is known as atrophic vaginitis. These vaginal changes may also make infections more common. Vaginal yeast infections and vaginitis are discussed on page 212.

The loss of moisture and lubrication in the vagina may lead to soreness during and after intercourse. However, vaginal changes do not have to lead to a decrease in sexual responsiveness or pleasure.

Mood Changes are caused by the hormonal and physical changes of menopause. Symptoms such as nervousness, lethargy, insomnia, moodiness, or depression are not uncommon.

With menopause, many women fear emotional upset and loss of sexuality. On the other hand, many women look forward to the freedom that menopause brings, particularly

Menopause - continued

freedom from the discomfort associated with the menstrual cycle and freedom from contraception.

Understanding what is happening to you and using home care techniques to relieve any discomfort will help you make the most of menopause.

Home Treatment

Irregular Periods

- Keep a written record of your periods--the date, length, the amount of flow--in case you need to confer with a health professional later.

Hot Flashes

- Keep your home and work place cool.

- Wear layers of loose clothing that can be easily removed.

- Drink lots of water and juices.

- Avoid caffeine and alcohol if they bring on hot flashes.

- Exercise regularly. This will help stabilize hormones and ease insomnia.

Vaginal Dryness

- Use a water-soluble vaginal lubricant such as K-Y Jelly or Surgilube. Vegetable oil will also work. Do not use a petroleum-based product such as Vaseline.

- Regular sexual activity (two to three times per week) improves circulation and suppleness in the vagina.

Mood Changes

- The best thing you can do for yourself is to realize you are not alone. Discuss your symptoms with other women. Give yourself, and ask from others, abundant amounts of love, caring, and understanding.

Birth Control during Menopause

Some women may continue to ovulate after menopause, which means there is a slight chance that they could become pregnant, even though they are no longer menstruating. Women who had their last period before age 50 and who do not want to become pregnant should continue using contraceptives (other than birth control pills) for two years. Women who had their last period after age 50 generally need to use contraceptives only for 12 months.

When to Call a Health Professional

- If you experience prolonged irregular bleeding, particularly if you are overweight.

- If vaginal dryness is unmanageable and not relieved by home treatment. Your doctor may prescribe estrogen that you can apply directly to the vagina as a cream or suppository.

- If you are considering estrogen replacement therapy (ERT). Estrogen therapy has been shown to reduce many of the symptoms of menopause as well as provide significant protection against heart disease and osteoporosis. However, ERT may increase a woman's risk of breast and uterine cancer. Knowing the facts, you can work in partnership with your physician to make the right decision for you.

Estrogen Replacement Therapy

Whether or not to take estrogen after menopause is a complex question. Estrogen replacement therapy reduces some health risks and increases others, and its overall impact on your health requires an evaluation of your individual health history and risk factors. The following factors may be important to your decision:

ERT and Osteoporosis

Estrogen replacement reduces the risk of osteoporosis by slowing bone loss and decreasing fracture rates. Currently, it is the only therapy that does so. It has been estimated that ERT can reduce the risk of osteoporotic fractures by up to 60 percent.

See page 51 to assess your risk for osteoporosis.

ERT and Heart Disease

Estrogen seems to protect against the development of heart disease, the leading cause of death in post-menopausal women. Primarily, ERT decreases "bad" low-density lipoprotein (LDL) cholesterol and increases "good" high-density lipoprotein (HDL) cholesterol levels. This particular combination lowers the risk of heart disease.

Because risk of death from cardiovascular disease is so much greater than other health risks for postmenopausal women, the "heart protection factor" of ERT may suggest that it is a wise choice for many women.

ERT and Breast Cancer

The jury is still out on ERT and increased risk of breast cancer. Some studies warn of increased risk. Other studies suggest that lower doses of estrogen do not appreciably increase risk of breast cancer even when administered over several years.

Women at high risk for breast cancer may decline ERT. If you do choose ERT, it is important to get a yearly mammogram.

ERT and Endometrial Cancer

ERT may increase the risk of endometrial cancer (cancer of the lining of the uterus). Estrogen combined with the hormone progestin seems to protect against this increased risk. On the other hand, adding progestin

ERT - continued

reduces the estrogen's ability to lower cholesterol levels. For more information on endometrial cancer, see page 214.

ERT and Other Considerations

Estrogen replacement greatly reduces discomfort caused by menopausal symptoms such as hot flashes, vaginal dryness, and mood swings. On the other hand, ERT may cause vaginal bleeding, weight gain, nausea, headaches, and breast tenderness.

ERT often requires daily administration. That means you have to remember to take a pill every day for as long as you continue the therapy.

Who Should *Not* Take ERT

If you have any of these conditions, ERT is generally not recommended:

- Diagnosed or suspected breast or endometrial (uterine) cancer

- Undiagnosed genital bleeding

- Active liver disease

- Active thromboembolic disease (blood clots)

Should *You* Take ERT?

Discuss each of the above risks and benefits with your doctor. The best ERT decision depends upon your individual risks. The following guidelines may also be helpful.

- The greater your risk of heart disease, the greater benefit you will receive from ERT. (If you have high cholesterol levels that you are unable to reduce, ERT may be very important to your health.)

- The greater your risk of osteoporosis, the greater benefit you will receive from ERT. (If you scored over 19 on the osteoporosis risk factor scale on page 51, ERT may be particularly valuable.)

- If you have low cholesterol and strong bones, you may feel that the benefits that you will gain from ERT are not worth the extra risks.

Vaginitis

Vaginitis is any vaginal infection, inflammation or irritation that causes a change in normal vaginal discharge. General symptoms include a marked change in the amount, color, odor or consistency of the discharge, itching, painful urination, and pain during intercourse.

Among older women, yeast infections are the most common kind of vaginitis. In addition to vaginal itching and painful urination, yeast infections cause a white, curdy "cottage cheese" discharge.

Post-menopausal women, who have lower estrogen levels, are more prone to vaginitis. Diabetes and the use of antibiotics or corticosteroids also increase risk.

Vaginitis is common and is not necessarily a symptom of a sexually transmitted disease. Some women seem more susceptible than others. An aggravating fact about vaginitis is that it can recur.

Prevention

- Wear cotton underpants. The organisms that cause vaginitis grow best in warm, moist places, and nylon underpants tend to trap heat and perspiration. Avoid clothing that is tight in the crotch and thighs.

- Wash your genital area once a day with a mild soap and warm water. Dry thoroughly.

- Avoid douching frequently. A healthy vagina will clean itself.

- Avoid feminine deodorant spray and other perfumed products. They irritate tender skin.

- Wipe from front to back after using the toilet to avoid spreading bacteria from the anus to the vagina.

- If you are taking antibiotics, include plenty of yogurt or buttermilk in your diet to help prevent a yeast infection.

Home Treatment

- A bacterial or non-specific infection may go away by itself in three to four days.

- Avoid intercourse to give irritated vaginal tissues time to heal.

- Avoid scratching. Relieve itching with cold water compresses.

- If you have burning and pain on urination, and feel the need to urinate frequently, see Urinary Tract Infection on page 115.

- Recurrent yeast infections may be treated with over-the-counter antifungal creams, Gyne-Lotrimin or Monistat.

When to Call a Health Professional

- If self-treatment fails to clear up a yeast infection within three to four days. Stronger medication may be prescribed.

Women's Cancers

Breast cancer, cervical cancer, endometrial cancer, and ovarian cancer account for 27 percent of all cancer deaths in women. Early detection and effective treatment have steadily increased the percentage of women who survive these forms of cancer.

The primary risk factors for each of these cancers are shown on page 216. If you have a family history of a particular cancer, or two or more other risk factors for any particular cancer, you may wish to increase your preventive measures and the frequency of regular exams.

Women's Cancers - continued

Breast Cancer

Apprcximately one out of every nine women will develop breast cancer. With improved detection and treatment methods, 90 percent of women survive at least five years after a diagnosis of breast cancer.

Early detection is important. Treatment options range from radiation and chemotherapy to lumpectomy or complete breast removal. Symptoms of breast cancer include:

- Lump, thickening, or swelling in the breast

- Dimpled skin (orange peel texture)

- Nipple discharge, scaliness, pain, or tenderness

Cervical Cancer

The cervix, or "neck of the womb," is a common site of cancer. Cervical cancer is easily detected by Pap tests. The five-year survival rate for all cervical cancer patients is 67 percent.

However, if the disease is discovered early, the rate is virtually 100 percent. Symptoms include:

- Vaginal bleeding not related to periods or menopause

- Abnormal vaginal discharge

Endometrial Cancer (Uterine Cancer)

Endometrial cancer affects the lining of the uterus. It is most common in women between the ages of 50 and 70. The overall five-year survival rate is 85 percent; 92 percent if discovered early, and almost 100 percent if found at the precancerous lesion stage. The primary symptom is vaginal bleeding not related to menopause.

Ovarian Cancer

Ovarian cancer is less common than the other women's cancers, but claims many lives because it is often not discovered until an advanced stage. The overall five-year survival rate is 38 percent. If found early, the survival rate improves to 85 percent. Ovarian cancer often presents no obvious symptoms until late in development. Then the symptoms include:

- Enlarged abdomen, caused by an accumulation of fluid

- Abnormal vaginal bleeding (rare)

- Stomach distention, gas, or discomfort

Home Treatment

- See "Winning Over Serious Illness" on page 311.

- Take good care of your mental health. Depression is a common response to a diagnosis of cancer.

Good home care can help you stay in a positive frame of mind, which will make your treatment as effective as possible. See page 242.

- Learn as much as you can about different treatment options. Work with your doctor to develop a treatment plan that will best meet your needs and desires. If you are not comfortable with the treatment options offered, consider a second opinion.

- If surgery is suggested, see page 13 for questions to ask your doctor.

When to Call a Health Professional

- If any symptom described above is not explained by other causes.

- If it is time for your routine breast or pelvic exam. Women with a family history of women's cancers or those with several other risk factors should schedule an annual breast and pelvic exam. Women who are not at high risk should follow the recommended schedule of exams on page 27.

Anyone with two or more risk factors for a particular cancer should increase preventive activities and the frequency of screening tests. See page 216 for risk factors.

Hysterectomy Guidelines

A hysterectomy is the surgical removal of the uterus. It is sometimes needed to save a life. However, it is too often performed unnecessarily. Hysterectomy is often the best solution for:

- Invasive endometrial or cervical cancer

- Ovarian cancer

- Large fibroids with severe bleeding and pain

- Severe prolapse of the uterus

- Severe and recurrent pelvic inflammatory disease (PID)

- Post-menopausal women with cervical cancer *in situ* or with severe uterine bleeding of unknown cause

Hysterectomy is generally not the best solution for:

- Cancer *in situ* for a premenopausal woman

- Fibroids with mild or no symptoms

- Endometriosis

- Prolapsed uterus that responds to exercise and other treatments

- Pelvic inflammatory disease that responds to other treatments

- Abnormal uterine bleeding

The general guidelines above may not apply to your case. Actively work with your doctor to decide if a hysterectomy is the best solution for your health problem.

Risk Factors for Women's Cancers

Risk Factor	Breast Cancer	Cervical Cancer	Endometrial Cancer	Ovarian Cancer
Family history (Mother, sister, or aunt)	✓	✓	✓	✓
Late menopause (after age 55)	✓		✓	
Early menopause (before age 45)				✓
No children or first child after age 30	✓		✓	✓
Endometrial cancer	✓			
Breast cancer			✓	
High animal fat diet*	✓			✓
Obesity*	✓		✓	
Menstruation before age 11	✓			
History of irregular periods			✓	
Intercourse before age 18		✓		
History of multiple sex partners		✓		
Herpes infections/ genital warts		✓		
History of infertility			✓	✓
Estrogen replacement Long-term or high-dose*	✓		✓	
Cigarette smoking*		✓		

Risks that can be changed

16

Men's Health

At first glance, men appear to be at a great disadvantage when it comes to life expectancy. Men have a much greater prevalence of heart disease, emphysema, cirrhosis, lung cancer, and fatal accidents. On average, women outlive men by seven years. In fact, by age 75, only two men are alive for every three women.

However, there is some good news lurking behind these facts. Nearly all the diseases that rob men of their years are self-inflicted. There is no hormonal cause for cigarette smoking, excessive alcohol consumption, sedentary lifestyle, or not using your seat belt. These are habits that can be unlearned the same way they were learned. If you can identify any life-shortening habits and work on developing healthy practices, you will likely add years to your life and surely add life to your years.

This chapter covers health problems that are of particular concern to men.

Baldness

Heredity is the biggest factor in determining when you will begin to lose your hair, but age comes in a strong second. By age 60, most men have some degree of baldness.

Hair loss can also be caused or accelerated by a variety of medications. These include some drugs for high blood pressure, high cholesterol, arthritis, and ulcers, as well as cancer chemotherapy.

Prevention

- Natural hair loss cannot be prevented.

- For medication-related hair loss, ask your physician if another drug may be substituted.

Baldness - continued

Home Treatment

- Baldness increases the risk of sunburn and skin cancer on the scalp. Wear a hat or use a sunscreen with a SPF of 15 or more.

When to Call a Health Professional

- If your hair loss is sudden, rather than gradual.

- If spots of baldness appear, rather than symmetrical, localized thinning.

- If there is a rash or scaliness associated with your hair loss.

- If you notice increased hair loss and you are taking medication for blood pressure, high cholesterol, arthritis, or ulcers. Ask your doctor or pharmacist if the medication could be the cause.

Erection Problems

As a man ages, the speed of his sexual response slows, his drive to reach orgasm is delayed, and the force of his orgasm gradually lessens. This is normal. These physical changes need not be seen as problems. In many cases, they can prolong sensual enjoyment prior to orgasm.

An erection problem, sometimes called impotence, is a persistent difficulty in achieving or maintaining an erection of the penis capable of intercourse. Note the word "persistent"; occasional episodes of impotence are perfectly normal and are nothing to worry about.

One out of every four men experiences a significant erection problem by age 65. However, it is not an inevitable part of getting older. There is no age limit to the ability of healthy men to have erections.

About half of all erection problems have at least some physical cause. Diabetes, heart and circulation problems, medication side effects, alcohol and drug abuse, and other physical problems contribute to impotence.

The other half can be traced to psychological factors, such as stress, anxiety, bereavement, depression, and negative feelings. Psychological and physical causes interact. Stress or anxiety will often combine with a minor physical problem to cause impotence.

Prevention

Erection problems can usually be prevented by taking a more relaxed approach to lovemaking and keeping a close watch for possible side effects from medications or illnesses.

Home Treatment

- Restrict alcohol. Even small amounts of alcohol can cause temporary impotence. Alcohol also reacts with many medications.

- Don't smoke. Smoking reduces blood flow, which can interfere with your ability to have an erection.

- Try for more foreplay. Let your partner know that you would enjoy more stroking. Slow down, then slow down some more.

- Relax. If you experience occasional bouts of impotence, worrying about how you will perform next time may only aggravate the problem.

- Consider your psychological concerns. If you are grieving over a loss, you may not be ready for erections during intercourse. Give yourself some time.

When to Call A Health Professional

- If you think that a medication may be causing the problem. Blood pressure medicines, diuretics, and mood-altering drugs are particularly troublesome. Check out the medicines you are now taking in the PDR (Physician's Desk Reference). Look to see if erection problems or impotence are listed as a side effect. See Resources Q1-3 on page 351 or ask your physician or pharmacist.

- If there is a loss of pubic or armpit hair and your breasts enlarge.

- If a few months of home treatment efforts have not brought relief, consider using the services of a psychological therapist. Therapy can be successful in about 80 percent of cases.

- If home treatment strategies have not worked after a few months, talk with your doctor about using a vacuum tumescent device. This suction pump mechanism can produce erections lasting up to 30 minutes.

- After all other options have been tried for several months without success, you may wish to talk with your doctor about penile implants or erection-producing medications.

Genital Health

Daily cleaning of the penis, particularly under the foreskin of an uncircumcised penis, can prevent bacterial infection and reduce the already low risk of penile cancer. Routine exams for genital health include a professional exam of the prostate every five years. Monthly testicular self-examinations have not been shown to be effective for men over 50.

Genital Health - continued

When to Call a Health Professional

- If you notice any lumps, nodules, or unexplained enlargement in the testicles.

- If you have unexplained groin pain.

- If you notice any penile discharge. Also see page 232.

Hernias

A hernia occurs when part of the intestine balloons out and protrudes into another part of the body. With an inguinal hernia, a part of the intestine protrudes down the inguinal canal into the scrotum. This condition is caused when exertion increases the pressure of the intestine against a congenitally weak spot in the abdominal wall. The exertion could be a result of heavy work, especially lifting, or even straining during bowel movements.

A hernia is called reducible if the bulge can be pushed back into place inside the abdomen; irreducible if it cannot.

Inguinal hernias can occur suddenly or gradually. Symptoms can include:

- A feeling of weakness or pressure in the groin

- Occasional pain or aches

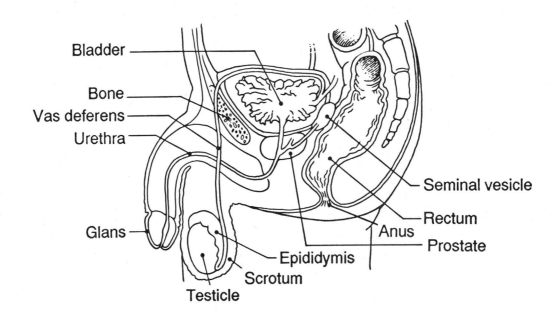

Male Genitals

- A gurgling feeling

- Visible bulges just above or within the scrotum. These bulges are easier to see if the person is coughing.

Strangulated hernias occur when irreducible hernias get so pinched that the blood supply is cut off and the tissue dies and swells. Rapidly worsening pain in and around the scrotum is a signal that the hernia is strangulated. The dead tissue quickly becomes infected and can lead to a life-threatening situation in a matter of hours.

Prevention

- Avoid activities that strain your abdominal area.

- Regularly work at keeping the muscles of the abdomen strong. Curl-ups (exercise #19 on page 274) are helpful.

- Avoid constipation. See page 99.

- If you lift heavy weights on a regular basis, consider wearing a weight-lifting belt to support the abdominal wall and prevent hernias.

Home Treatment

- Follow the advice in the prevention section.

- Pay close attention to increasing pain or other signs of a strangulated hernia.

When to Call a Health Professional

- If you suspect a hernia, you should see your physician for a full diagnosis and evaluation of the risk.

- If you experience progressive abdominal or scrotal pain.

- If mild groin pain continues for more than one week.

Prostate Problems

The prostate is a doughnut-shaped cluster of glands that lies at the bottom of the bladder, about halfway between the rectum and the base of the penis. It encircles the urethra, the tube that carries urine from the bladder out through the penis. This walnut-sized gland produces some of the fluid that transports sperm during ejaculation.

The three most common prostate problems for older men are: infections (prostatitis), prostate enlargement (benign prostatic hypertrophy), and prostate cancer.

Prostatitis *(Prostate Infection)*
There are two types of prostate infection--chronic and acute. **Chronic prostatitis** frequently accompanies a urinary tract infection and shares those symptoms:

- Pain and burning on urination and ejaculation

Prostate Problems - continued

- A strong and frequent urge to urinate while passing only small amounts of urine

- Blood in the urine (occasionally)

Acute prostatitis comes on suddenly with the additional symptoms of fever, chills, and back or abdominal pain.

Prostate infections will usually respond well to home care and antibiotic therapy. In some cases, the infection will recur every few weeks. Long-term treatment with antibiotics may be necessary.

Prevention

- Avoid alcohol, coffee, tea, and spicy foods.

- Drink more fluids, both water and fruit juices. Extra fluids help flush the urinary tract clean. Try to drink three quarts a day.

- Keep stress under control. A high level of stress is closely associated with these infections.

Home Treatment

- Drink as much water as you can tolerate.

- Hot baths help soothe pain and reduce stress.

- Eliminate all alcohol, coffee, tea, and spicy foods from your diet.

When to Call a Health Professional

- If urinary symptoms are combined with fever, chills, vomiting, or pain in the back or abdomen.

- If symptoms continue for seven days despite home care.

- If there is blood in the urine.

- If you have urinary or ejaculatory pain and a discharge from your penis.

Prostate Enlargement *(Benign Prostatic Hypertrophy)*

By age 65, virtually every man's prostate has enlarged. As the gland swells, it tends to squeeze the urethra and cause urinary problems. Men with enlarged prostates may notice:

- Difficulty in getting urine started and completely stopped (dribbling)

- The urge to urinate frequently

- Decreased force of urine stream

- Incomplete emptying of the bladder

An enlarged prostate gland is not a serious problem unless urination becomes extremely difficult or backed-up urine causes bladder infections or kidney damage.

Surgery is usually not necessary for an enlarged prostate. Although it used to be a common treatment for benign prostatic hypertrophy, it has recently been found that most cases do not get worse over time as previously thought. Many men find that their symptoms are stable and some even clear up on their own. In these cases, the best treatment may be no treatment at all.

Unless the prostate continues to enlarge and causes bladder and kidney infections, surgery is probably not needed. Your doctor can advise you on the various treatment options. Some recent progress has been made in the development of drugs which improve symptoms without surgery.

Prevention

- Since the prostate produces seminal fluid, a long-standing belief exists that regular ejaculations (two to three times per week) will help prevent an enlarged prostate. There is no scientific evidence of this, but it is without risk.

- The prostate gland can be felt by a health professional during a rectal examination. Exams are recommended every five years after age 50.

Home Treatment

- Avoid antihistamines and decongestants. These drugs can contribute to urine retention.

- If you are bothered by a frequent need to urinate at night, cut down on beverages, especially alcohol and caffeine, before bedtime.

- Don't postpone urinating, and take plenty of time. Try sitting on the toilet instead of standing.

- If dribbling after urination is a problem, wash your penis once a day.

When to Call a Health Professional

- If fever, chills, or abdominal pain develop.

- Diuretics, tranquilizers, antihistamines, and anti-depressants can aggravate urinary problems. If you take these drugs, ask your health professional if there are alternative medications without these side effects.

- Make an appointment to see your health professional if the symptoms of an enlarged prostate last longer than two weeks. Early examination enables you to be sure of the diagnosis and consider treatment options.

Prostate Cancer

Most men who have prostate cancer will never know it. The cancer is slow-growing, and they will die of other diseases before it has caused any symptoms.

Prostate cancer and prostate enlargement (benign prostatic hypertrophy) have similar symptoms, but the two

Prostate Cancer - continued

conditions are not related. Enlargement of the prostate does not cause cancer. The symptoms of prostate cancer include:

- Decreased strength of the urine stream

- Difficulty getting urine started or completely stopped (dribbling)

- Frequent and painful urination

- Hip or lower back pain

- Blood or pus in the urine

Prostate cancer is the second leading cause of cancer deaths in men in the U.S. When detected early, before it has spread into the bones and other body tissues, prostate cancer is generally curable, and survival rates are good. Prostate cancer is usually detected by a doctor's rectal exam. There are other detection methods, including a blood test (prostate-specific antigen, or PSA) and ultrasound.

The most important risk factor for prostate cancer is family history. If your father, brothers, uncles, or grandfathers have had prostate cancer, consider more frequent rectal exams. Other risk factors include smoking and a high-fat diet.

Prevention

- Avoid smoking and other tobacco use. Smokers have a 20 percent greater risk of developing prostate cancer and a 50 percent greater chance of dying from it.

- Reduce the fat in your diet. See page 285 for suggestions.

- Consider a diet high in zinc. This important trace mineral is found in milk, whole grains, peas, carrots, and oysters.

Home Treatment

- Report any unusual urinary symptoms to your doctor, especially if they occur with back or hip pain.

- Learn all you can about the choices for treating prostate cancer. Sometimes a watchful waiting approach is best, especially if the cancer is in an early stage and is not causing symptoms. Because the cancer is slow-growing, regular monitoring will allow you and your doctor to decide when and if more aggressive treatment is needed. A treatment decision will depend on the stage of the cancer and your overall health.

- See Winning Over Serious Illness on page 311.

When to Call a Health Professional

- If any of the above described symptoms continue longer than two weeks.

- For a routine rectal/prostate exam. Early detection of prostate cancer usually ensures successful treatment. However, experts disagree on how often you should schedule rectal/prostate exams. You and your doctor can decide on an appropriate schedule for you. You may want to consider the following guidelines.

  - If you have a family history of prostate cancer, smoke, or have a high-fat diet, schedule an annual rectal exam.

  - If you have no risk factors, schedule a rectal exam every five years.

*Age may well offer the opportunity to understand sex
as intimate communication in its finest sense.*
Norman M. Lobsenz

17

Sexual Health

Sex and sexuality communicate a great deal: affection, love, esteem, warmth, sharing, and bonding. These gifts are as much the birthright of those in their 80s and 90s as those much younger.

Three aspects of sexuality are covered in this chapter: the changes that come with aging, suggestions on how to adjust to these changes, and information on sexual health problems.

Sexuality and Physical Changes with Aging

In most healthy adults, pleasure and interest in sex do not diminish with aging. Age alone is no reason to change the sexual practices that you have enjoyed throughout your life. However, sexual response does slow down as you age and you may have to make a few minor adjustments.

Common Physical Changes in Men

- It may take longer to get an erection and more time needs to pass between erections.

- Erections may be less firm with age. For information on erection problems, see page 218.

- Older men are able to delay ejaculation for a longer time.

Common Physical Changes in Women

Most physical changes take place after menopause and are due to lower estrogen levels.

- It may take longer to become sexually excited.

- Skin may feel more sensitive and irritable, making caressing and skin-to-skin contact less pleasurable.

Physical Changes - continued

- The walls of the vagina become thinner, drier, and more easily irritated during intercourse. (Use vaginal cream or K-Y Jelly to reduce the irritation. Your doctor can also prescribe a vaginal cream containing estrogen, which will help reverse the changes in the vaginal tissues.)

- Orgasms may be somewhat shorter than they used to be.

- Contractions experienced during orgasm can be uncomfortable.

Sexuality and Cultural and Psychological Changes

In addition to physical changes that affect sexuality in later years, there are cultural and psychological factors, too. Take ageism, for example. In our culture, sexuality is equated with youthful looks and youthful vigor. Too many people seem to think that as a person ages, he or she becomes less desirable and less of a sexual being. Older adults may accept this stereotype and buy into the notion that they are not permitted or expected to be sexual.

Joy in sex and loving knows no age barriers. Almost everyone has the capacity to find lifelong pleasure in sex. To believe in the myth that "old people have no interest in sex" is to miss out on wonderful possibilities.

Being single through choice, divorce, or widowhood can present a problem as well. By age 60, there are five single women for every single man, and that ratio goes up with increasing years. Women and men who are single may not know how to deal with their sexual feelings. Generally speaking, it is better to take some risks and express your desires than to suppress them until you are no longer aware that they exist.

Physical and emotional needs change with time and circumstance. Intimacy and sexuality may or may not be important to you. The issue here is one of choice. If you freely decide that sex is no longer right for you, then that is the correct decision. It is possible to live a fulfilling life without sex. However, if you choose to continue enjoying your sexuality, you deserve support and encouragement. You may find uncharted sensual territories left to explore.

Use It or Lose It: Keeping Sexual

Just as exercise is the key to maintaining fitness, sex on a regular basis is the best way to maintain sexual capacity. On the other hand, it is never too late to get started. Many older people who had been celibate for years have developed satisfying sexual practices within new loving relationships. For others, self-stimulation is common and poses no health risks or side effects.

Other considerations:

- To enhance sexual response, use more foreplay and direct contact with sexual organs.

- The mind is an erogenous zone. Fantasy and imagination help arouse some people.

- Many medications, especially antihypertensives, tranquilizers, and some heart medications, inhibit sexual response. Check with your doctor about lower doses or alternative medications.

- Colostomies, mastectomies, and other operations that involve changes in physical appearance need not put an end to sexual activities. A little counseling for both partners can help them adjust.

- People with heart conditions can enjoy full, satisfying sexual lives. Most physicians recommend only a brief period of abstention following a heart attack. Ask your doctor.

- If arthritis keeps you from enjoying sex, experiment with different positions and try using cushions below the hips. Also work to alleviate arthritis pain. See page 32.

- Drink alcohol only in moderation. Small amounts may heighten sexual responsiveness by squelching inhibitions, but larger amounts play havoc with your body.

Other Aspects of Sexuality

Sexuality goes far beyond the physical act itself. It is part of who we are. It involves our needs for touch, affection, and intimacy.

Touch

Touch is a wonderful and needed sense. Babies who are not touched do not thrive. Children who are not touched develop emotional problems. Touch is important to older adults as well. Touch adds to our sexuality; it helps us to feel connected with others.

- Get a massage. Professional massages are wonderful, but simple shoulder and neck rubs feel great, too. Find a friend who will trade shoulder rubs with you. See page 301 for instructions.

- Look for hugs. Everybody needs them. Some people are a little shy about hugs, but it's okay to ask, "Would you like a hug?" Many cultures use hugs instead of handshakes, and for good reason.

- Consider getting a pet. Caring for a pet can help meet your needs for touch. Some studies have shown that older people who are given pets to care for live longer.

Affection

To give and receive affection is a wonderful feeling. If you like someone, be sure to let them know. If someone seems to like you,

Sexuality - continued

appreciate it. It is never too late to make new friends and to strengthen bonds with longtime companions.

Intimacy

Intimacy is the capacity for a close physical or emotional connection with another person. Intimacy is a great protector against depression.

Talking with a confidant helps to ease life's problems. When someone loses a loved one, intimacy may be what is most missed. You can begin to rebuild intimacy in your life in the following ways:

- Turn to your children, siblings, or old and new friends.

- Look for another in your same situation. One of the richest benefits from support groups is that members often find intimacy with one another.

- Be available to others. Just as you need people, there are people who need you, too.

Sexual Health Problems

Sexually transmitted diseases (STD) or venereal diseases (VD) are infections passed from person to person through sexual intercourse or genital contact. AIDS, chlamydia, gonorrhea, syphilis, genital herpes, and genital warts are all STDs.

AIDS

About ten percent of the AIDS (acquired immunodeficiency syndrome) cases reported in the United States involve people aged 50 and over. AIDS is caused by the human immunodeficiency virus (HIV).

A person who has been exposed to the virus is said to be HIV-positive if antibodies to the virus are detected in the blood. It may take up to three months after infection for the antibodies to appear. Once active, the virus reduces the immune system's ability to fight infectious diseases. People with AIDS are at higher risk for other illnesses or cancers.

AIDS spreads when blood, semen, or other body fluids from an infected person enter the body of someone else. AIDS is not easy to catch. AIDS is not spread by mosquito bites, dirty toilets, being coughed on by an infected person, or touching someone with the disease.

Specific behaviors that spread AIDS include (from most risky to least risky):

1. Sharing injection needles and syringes with someone who is HIV-positive.

2. Rectal entry (anal) intercourse with someone who is HIV-positive. Rectal entry sex often tears the rectal blood vessels. This

allows AIDS transmissions to occur.

3. Unprotected sexual intercourse with someone who is HIV-positive.

4. Receiving blood transfusions, blood products, or organs donated by someone who is HIV-positive. Because all blood and blood products are now tested for the HIV virus, the risk of getting AIDS from blood transfusions is very low. However, someone who received a blood transfusion between 1977 and 1985 could have been infected.

A person who has been infected may not develop symptoms of AIDS for up to 10 years or longer, even though his or her body has produced antibodies to the virus. When AIDS does develop, the symptoms will vary according to which illnesses the reduced immunity has allowed to develop. Common symptoms are:

- Extreme fatigue

- Rapid weight loss

- Increased bruising

- Repeated diarrhea

- Recurring fevers and night sweats

- Swelling of glands in the neck and armpits

- Deep dry cough

- Shortness of breath

- Whitish color on tongue

- Unexplained bleeding from growths on the skin

- A personality change or mental deterioration

Each of these symptoms can be caused by many illnesses other than AIDS. If any symptom develops without a good explanation, call your doctor.

A simple blood test can determine if you are HIV-positive. While a positive test does not mean that you will get AIDS, it does mean that you are capable of transmitting the AIDS virus.

Prevention

- Avoid unprotected intercourse with anyone who may have had other sex partners or may have shared needles for drug use anytime since 1979.

- Insist on using condoms with any sex partner whose sexual history you do not know to be risk-free.

- Never share needles or syringes.

- Do not share toothbrushes, razors, tattoo needles, or other personal devices that could be contaminated with blood.

- For more information, call the National AIDS Hotline at 1-800-342-AIDS.

Sexually Transmitted Diseases

Chlamydia (kla-mid-ee-uh) is a disease that infects millions of men and women each year. Mild symptoms include vaginal discharge, stomach pain, and pain on urination.

If untreated, pelvic inflammatory disease may occur. Men may have some penile discharge and painful urination.

Gonorrhea is caused by bacteria spread through intimate contact. Symptoms include painful urination with vaginal discharge or a thick discharge from the penis. Many people have the bacteria but have no noticeable symptoms.

Genital herpes is caused by a virus that is easily spread through sexual contact and other direct skin contact. Symptoms occur two to thirty days after contact with an infected person.

The first symptoms include itching, burning, or tingling sensations in the genitals. Afterward, sores and blisters will appear on the genitals. Once infected, you may suffer from recurrent outbreaks. Some people have the virus but do not have any symptoms.

Genital warts are caused by a virus. In women, the warts may appear on the vagina, the cervix, or around the anus. Warts on the cervix are usually detected by a Pap smear. See page 208. Genital warts in men are usually found on the penis or scrotum. All genital warts need to be removed by a health professional.

Women who have had genital herpes or genital warts are at higher risk for cervical cancer. See page 216, "Risk Factors for Women's Cancers."

Syphilis is a bacterial infection that is spread through sexual contact. Symptoms appear two weeks to one month after contact. The first symptom is a small red blister or pimple on the genitals, called a chancre, which may go unnoticed. The lymph nodes in the groin may also swell.

If syphilis is not treated early, it can proceed to a second phase. Symptoms of the second phase can include headaches, bone pain, skin rashes, hair loss, and other symptoms that are easily confused with other illnesses.

Prevention

Preventing a sexually transmitted disease is easier than treating an infection once it occurs.

- Use condoms with any new partner until you are certain that person does not have any sexually transmitted diseases. Remember that it can take up to three months for antibodies to the HIV virus to develop and be detected in the blood.

- Avoid all intimate and sexual contact with anyone who has symptoms of an STD or who has been exposed to an STD. Keep in mind that many people do not have any symptoms, but can still transmit the disease to you. Condoms will help prevent you from contracting an STD from a person who has no visible symptoms.

- If you or your partner has herpes, avoid sexual contact when a blister is present, and use condoms at all other times.

When to Call a Health Professional

All STDs need to be diagnosed and treated by a health professional. Venereal disease clinics and public health agencies can provide STD diagnosis and treatment for a low cost. If you notice any unusual discharge or sores, or if you suspect that you have been exposed, make an appointment as soon as possible.

*To be seventy years young
is sometimes far more cheerful and hopeful
than to be forty years old.*
Oliver Wendell Holmes on the
70th birthday of Julia Ward Howe

18

Mental Self-Care

Mental health problems are pretty much the same as other health problems: everybody has to deal with them; most are quite minor and respond well to home treatment; and there are basic guidelines to follow when professional help is needed.

Increasingly, medical science is discovering that mental health problems often have a physical cause. Psychological problems are no longer thought of as weaknesses of character. Instead, we now know that the cause of mental health problems is complex. Often these problems begin when environmental or psychological stress triggers chemical imbalances in the brain. While some people can withstand more stress than others, nobody is immune to mental illness, once the stress reaches his or her limits.

Because the cause of mental health problems is both physical and psychological, both self-care and professional care are often needed.

The goal is to reduce the stress and to restore chemical balance in the brain.

Good mental self-care requires a keen awareness and understanding of symptoms. If you can recognize symptoms early and address the underlying causes, you can often prevent major mental health problems. Early recognition of symptoms can also allow you to seek help to resolve the problem before serious disruptions in your life occur.

Seeking Professional Help

Go in search of professional help when:

- A symptom becomes severe or disruptive.

- A disruptive symptom becomes a continuous or permanent pattern of behavior and does not respond to self-care efforts.

Professional Help - continued

- Symptoms become numerous and pervasive in all areas of a person's life and do not respond to self-care or communication efforts.

There is a wide range of professional and lay resources to choose from for mental health problems. Here are a few:

The Family Doctor: Mental health problems often have physical causes. Your physician can review your medications and medical history for clues. He or she can then refer you to other appropriate resources.

Psychiatrists: A psychiatrist is a physician who specializes in mental disorders. Psychiatrists can prescribe medications and order medical treatments. They also counsel patients.

Psychologists, social workers, and counselors: These professionals receive special training in helping people deal with mental health problems. They help patients identify, understand, and work through disturbing thoughts and emotions.

Pastors: People often turn to their clergy for counseling and advice in times of emotional distress. Many pastors have formal training in counseling. Many do not.

Cost Management Tips

The old saying, "talk is cheap," does not apply to most professional psychotherapists and counselors. The following tips can help keep costs down.

- Avoid just picking a name from the Yellow Pages. Talk with people you trust for a good referral.

- Use mental health professionals to help you identify the real problem and develop a self-management plan to resolve it.

- Emphasize the importance of self-care in the treatment plan.

- Ask about group therapy options.

- Cultivate special friends, join support groups, or look for peer counseling opportunities. Understanding and acceptance can help you to resolve the problem.

- Check out 12-step programs such as Alcoholics Anonymous, Al-Anon, Overeaters Anonymous, and other groups that can help you deal with the problem. Such programs are usually free, effective, and available in most communities.

Alcohol Problems

A person has an alcohol problem if his or her use of alcohol interferes with health or daily functioning. A person develops alcoholism if he or she becomes physically or psychologically dependent on alcohol.

The cause of alcoholism seems to be a combination of genetics and human behavior. Some people, especially the children of alcoholics, are genetically at a somewhat higher risk for alcoholism. Once alcohol dependency develops, it becomes very difficult to abstain without outside help. Medical detoxification may be needed.

For older adults, it is important to remember that:

- Alcohol slows down brain activity.

- Alcohol impairs mental alertness, memory, judgment, physical coordination, and reaction time.

- Alcohol increases the risk of falls and accidents.

- Heavy use of alcohol can cause permanent damage to the brain, central nervous system, liver, heart, kidneys, and stomach.

- Heavy alcohol use can lead to loss of employment, friends, and loved ones.

Aging also increases risks for these alcohol-related problems:

- Alcohol stays in the body longer as you age and tolerance for it decreases. Drinking the same amount that you drank 20 years ago can cause a lot more damage.

- Alcohol complicates many medical problems.

- Tranquilizers, barbiturates, certain painkillers, and antihistamines all increase the intoxicating effect of alcohol.

- Alcohol interferes with the medical benefits of many drugs, including anticonvulsants, anticoagulants, and diabetic medications. Alcohol combined with diuretics causes dizziness.

Screening Test

Many people will deny that they have an alcohol problem. The following questions may help you, or others, recognize an alcohol problem.

- Have you felt the need to cut down on your drinking?

- Are you annoyed by references to your drinking?

- Do you ever feel guilty about your drinking or hide it from others?

- Do you ever feel the need for an early morning drink?

A positive answer to two or more questions raises the possibility of an alcohol problem and the need for outside help.

Alcohol Problems - continued

Prevention

- Recognize the importance of cutting back on alcohol as you age.

- Seek friendships with people who do not rely on alcohol to enjoy themselves.

- Stay active and maintain daily responsibilities.

- Maintain social contacts with people following any major loss or life change.

- Be particularly cautious in your drinking if your parents or grandparents had alcohol problems.

Home Treatment

- Review the prevention guidelines above.

- Recognize early signs that alcohol use is becoming a problem.

- Look for other signs of mental stress. Try to understand and resolve sources of depression, anxiety, or loneliness.

- Attend an Alcoholics Anonymous meeting.

- If you are concerned about another person's alcohol use:

  - Build up his self-esteem.

  - Do not attack his morals. Be non-judgmental.

  - Never ignore the problem. Ask about it. Talk about it. Just don't nag about it.

  - Avoid scare tactics such as, "You're killing yourself." Discuss it as a medical problem.

  - Ask if he would accept help. Don't give up after the first "no." Keep asking. If he ever agrees, act that very day to arrange for help. Call a health professional or Alcoholics Anonymous for an immediate appointment. See Resources C1-2 on page 349.

  - Attend a meeting of Al-Anon.

When to Call a Health Professional

- If you recognize an alcohol problem and are ready to accept help. Look for a professional with experience in alcohol-related problems.

Anger/Hostility

Anger acts as a signal to your body to prepare for a fight. General hostility is remaining ready for a fight all the time.

When you become angry, adrenaline and other hormones are released into your blood stream and your blood pressure goes up. Continual hostility increases your risk for heart attack and other illnesses. It can also isolate you from other people.

Home Treatment

- Notice when you first get angry. Don't ignore your anger until it erupts.

- Identify the real cause of the anger.

- Express your anger in a safe way.

  ○ Talk about it with a friend.

  ○ Draw or paint to release the anger.

  ○ Try screaming or yelling in a private place.

  ○ Write daily in a journal.

- Count to ten. Give yourself a little time for your adrenaline level to go down.

- Use "I" statements, not "you" statements, to discuss your anger. Say "I feel angry when your plans do not consider my needs," instead of "You make me mad when you are so inconsiderate."

- Forgive and forget. Forgiving helps lower blood pressure and eases your muscle tension. You will feel more relaxed.

- Books on anger can help. See Resources E1-2 on page 349.

When to Call a Health Professional

- If hostility has or could result in violence or harm to yourself or someone else.

- If anger or hostility interferes with your work, home, or friends.

- Also see Seeking Professional Help on page 235.

Anxiety

Anxiety is the presence of an undefined fear without an obvious or immediate source of danger. A disorder occurs when anxiety symptoms become overwhelming and interfere with daily life.

The symptoms of anxiety are divided into two categories:

Physical Symptoms

- Trembling, twitching, or shaking

- Muscle tension, aches, or soreness

- Restlessness

- Fatigue

- Breathlessness

- Pounding heart

- Sweating

- Cold, clammy hands

- Dry mouth

- Dizziness or lightheadedness

Anxiety - continued

- Chills or hot flashes

- Frequent urination or diarrhea

- Nausea

Emotional Symptoms

- Apprehension

- Excessive worrying

- Feeling that something bad is going to happen

- Poor concentration

- Excessive startle response

- Insomnia

- Irritability or agitation

- Depression

Anxiety from specific situations or fears can cause any or all of these symptoms for a short time. When the frightening situation is over, the symptoms subside. Many people develop generalized anxiety disorders in which many of the symptoms remain even when there is no identifiable cause. Home treatment combined with medical care can be very effective.

Home Treatment

- Recognize and accept anxiety about specific fears or situations. Say to yourself, "Okay, I see the problem. Now I'll start to deal with it."

- Notice and track your anxiety symptoms and talk about them with a friend. Anxiety decreases when you objectively analyze the situation and consider your options.

- Force yourself to go ahead in spite of your fears.

- Consider whether caffeine, medications, delirium, or dementia might be making you anxious.

- Develop positive expectations for the future.

- Reading about anxiety control can help. See Resources F1-2 on page 349.

When to Call a Health Professional

- If you regularly experience anxiety symptoms.

- If you are unable to break out of a state of anxiety by using home treatment alone.

- If you are concerned that hyperthyroidism (see page 126) may be causing the anxiety symptoms.

Depression

At some point in their lives, most people experience some form of depression. Depression can range from a minor problem to a major life-threatening illness. Depression is treatable. For many people, effective treatment can mean a whole new life.

Medical science is getting closer to understanding depression. Most major depressions involve an imbalance of neurotransmitters (chemical messengers that stimulate different functions in the brain). An imbalance in these brain chemicals can be triggered by many things:

- A loss of a loved one or something that is highly valued

- Chronic stress or a stressful event

- A major illness

- Reactions to many medications

- Alcoholism, drug abuse, dementia, and other mental health problems

- A reduction of intense light during winter seems to cause a form of depression called seasonal affective disorder in some people (see page 242)

Some people are genetically susceptible to chemical imbalances in the brain. For these and others at high risk for depression, it is fortunate that effective treatments are available.

Sad feelings do not always mean that you are heading for a major depression. Bad news or disappointment can cause you to feel sad--perhaps for several days without relief. This is normal and healthy as long as you don't get stuck in those sad feelings. Grief can also cause a normal sadness. See page 245.

Everyone gets sad. Gauging how deep and pervasive your sad feelings are can help you decide what you should do. See "Normal Sadness or Depression?" on page 243 to help determine if you are suffering from depression.

Caregiver Tips for Depression

- Help the person to rebuild self-esteem. Help him remember the positive things he has done and good times he has had.

- Help the person to feel more in control of his situation.

- Encourage activity with others.

- Depressed people can lose objectivity about themselves. If signs of major depression are strong, insist that the person talk with a mental health professional.

- Caregivers get depressed too. If you start to feel depressed, use the home treatment tips to get back on track.

- Remember that depression can often mimic dementia. Try to rule out depression if the person seems confused, withdrawn, or has other symptoms that appear to be dementia.

Depression - continued

Home Treatment

No matter how depressed you are, you can get back to normal. Self-care may be enough to pull you out of a mild depression. For more serious depression, self-care can add to the benefits of professional treatment.

- At the first sign of sadness or depression, ask a friend for some extra attention. You can lose objectivity about yourself when you're feeling blue.

- Consider what might be causing or adding to your sad feelings:

  o Is it drug-induced? Review your prescription and over-the-counter medications with a pharmacist or physician.

  o If it's winter time or you have not seen much sunshine in a while, read the information about seasonal affective disorder on this page.

- Keep on going. It is easier to **do** yourself into **feeling** better than to **feel** yourself into **doing** better.

- Get regular exercise. If nothing else, go for long walks. They help to clear the mind.

- Look for a laugh. Laughter, like exercise, can help restore balance to your system.

Seasonal Affective Disorder (Winter Depression)

There is increasing evidence (not yet conclusive) that a lack of sunlight during winter months can cause depression in some people. Symptoms include melancholy moods, changes in sleeping habits, cravings for sweets and starchy foods, and chronic tiredness. If you notice such a pattern developing during the winter, consider the following:

- When the winter sun does shine, go outside and soak it up. (Protect your skin--it is the eye's exposure to sunlight that makes the difference.)

- Go south for a winter vacation, if you can.

- Some people may benefit from light therapy. They sit in front of bright, full-spectrum fluorescent lights for one to five hours a day. They often notice improvement by the end of the first week of daily treatments.

  Because it is still a new approach to winter depression, the National Institutes of Health recommend that light therapy be supervised by a health professional.

- Work on ways to boost your self-esteem. Read the Mental Wellness Chapter beginning on page 305.

- Tell yourself that this mood will pass. Then, look for signs that it is ending.

- Surround yourself with happy, upbeat people.

- Books can help. See Resources K1-2 on page 350.

When to Call a Health Professional

Health professionals can do a great deal to help you break out of depression. There are three general forms of treatment: counseling (psychotherapy), medication, and electroconvulsive therapy (ECT).

Counseling and medication are often used together. Because many things can contribute to depression, combining different self-care and professional treatments is often most helpful.

ECT is the least common approach for treating depression. It is usually used only for dealing with a major depression. In such cases, it can be of great value.

All three methods can be effective in restoring chemical balance to your brain and emotional well-being to your life. Try self-care first, but if any of the following statements apply, call your doctor or a mental health professional:

Normal Sadness or Depression?

If you have experienced four or more of the following symptoms nearly every day for more than two weeks, you may be suffering from depression:

- Feelings of sadness, anxiety, or hopelessness

- Lack of interest or pleasure in usual activities and pastimes

- Increase or decrease in appetite; or unexplained gain or loss of weight

- Frequent backaches, headaches, stomach troubles, or other aches that don't respond to treatment

- Insomnia or excessive sleepiness

- Low energy, fatigue, tiredness

- Feeling restless or irritable

- Feeling worthless or guilty

- Inability to concentrate, remember, or make decisions

- Frequent thoughts of suicide or death

Home treatment (see page 242) may be all that is needed for mild cases. However, if home treatment doesn't help lift your mood within two weeks, contact a health professional. Counseling and medication, combined with your continued home treatment, can successfully deal with most cases of depression.

Depression - continued

- You suspect you are very depressed. See "Normal Sadness or Depression?" on page 243.

- You suspect you are depressed and two weeks of home treatment has not helped.

- You are feeling suicidal.

Drug Abuse

Most people think of drug abuse as the illegal use of marijuana, cocaine, heroin, or other "street" drugs. Drug abuse among older adults is more likely to be drug "misuse"--the unintentional overuse of legal prescription drugs.

Tranquilizers, sedatives, painkillers, and amphetamines are often misused unintentionally or accidentally. Older women are at particular risk; over two-thirds of all prescriptions for tranquilizers are written for women.

The symptoms of drug misuse vary widely, depending upon the kind of drug. Often, they occur slowly over a long period of time, and can be confused with symptoms of other health problems.

See page 340 for a list of symptoms that may be caused by adverse drug reactions.

Drug dependence or addiction occurs when you develop a physical or psychological "need" for a drug. You may not be aware that you have become dependent on a drug until you try to stop taking it suddenly. Withdrawing from the drug can produce uncomfortable symptoms. The usual treatment is to gradually reduce the dose of the drug until it can be stopped completely.

Prevention

- Do not regularly use medications to sleep, lose weight, or relax without careful supervision by your doctor. Look for non-drug solutions.

- Carefully follow the instructions for taking tranquilizers, sedatives, painkillers, and antidepressants. If your doctor prescribes these drugs, ask to start at the lowest dose possible. If you are already taking them, see if it is possible to slowly reduce the dose.

- Do not suddenly stop taking any medication without your doctor's supervision. Serious symptoms can result if some medications are abruptly withdrawn.

- Do not take any medications with alcohol. Alcohol can react with many medications and cause serious complications.

Home Treatment

The best home treatment for drug misuse is to stay alert for early signs that adverse drug reactions or dependency are developing.

- Ask your pharmacist if any of your current medications could potentially lead to overuse problems.

- Be especially cautious of the following types of medications:

  o Painkillers (Codeine, Darvon, Demerol, Percodan, and others)

  o Tranquilizers (Ativan, Librium, Valium, and other benzodiazepines)

  o Sedatives/Sleeping Pills (Seconal, Phenobarbital, Nembutal, and other barbiturates plus Dalmane, Doriden, Halcion, other nonbarbiturates, and over-the-counter sleep aids)

- Discuss with your doctor all medications you are taking, including over-the-counter products. Gradually reduce the dosages of any that you agree are not needed.

- See Chapter 25, Medication Management, for tips on how to take your medications correctly and avoid adverse reactions.

When to Call a Health Professional

- Anytime you suspect that you or someone you know is becoming dependent on or misusing a medication. You will need a doctor's help to reduce the dosage or to stop taking the drug.

Illegal Drugs

As the average age of the general population goes up, we will find more illegal drug use among older adults. It is important to remember that normal changes that come with aging affect how drugs, both legal and illegal, are processed by the body. The health risks of illegal drugs could be even greater for older adults. If you want help, look under "Drug Abuse" in your local Yellow Pages.

Grief

Grief is a natural healing process that enables a person to adjust to significant change or loss. Although painful, grief is also of great benefit. It provides a period of adjustment and an opportunity to build a foundation for a meaningful future.

Grief can be expressed physically as well as emotionally. Physical symptoms include sighing, exhaustion, insomnia, restlessness, constipation, diarrhea, and nausea. Emotional responses to loss can consist of denial, anger, guilt, depression, and many other strong feelings.

It is not uncommon to be preoccupied with the image of a loved one who has died. Survivors often report seeing, having conversations with, or even being touched by the deceased person. This is normal.

Grief - continued

No person or book can tell you what your grief "should" be like. How long and in what ways you grieve will be unique to you. There are, however, stages of grief that are more or less common to many who suffer a loss.

The Stages of Grief

Grief is different for everyone. Your grief may not progress directly from one stage to the next. However, understanding what others have experienced can help you deal with your own emotions.

Shock and Denial: The "Not Me" Stage

If your loss is sudden, your first reaction may be shock. Shock is a natural anesthesia that protects you from overwhelming pain. You may even act as if nothing has happened. You may feel numb. Later, you may not remember how you felt or acted during this period.

Denial is normal. You understand what has happened, but on a deeper level you don't really believe it.

Denial may pass quickly, or last for months or even years. Denial is all right for a while. It provides a brief respite before you have to gear up to deal with the loss. However, if denial lasts too long, it may separate the grieving person from reality.

Tips for Caregivers

At every stage of the grieving process, caregivers and friends can provide valuable support.

Shock/Denial Stage

- Give hugs, hold hands. Send cards, notes, flowers.
- Provide food, transportation.
- Do chores but expect the person to help, too.
- Help the person to see the evidence of the loss.
- Give the person time alone.

Guilt/Anger Stage

- Listen, listen, listen. Show no judgment unless asked.
- Call or visit often. Be together in silence.
- Accept abrupt mood shifts.
- Provide assurance that the person was not to blame.
- Recommend and help arrange for support groups.

Adjustment/Acceptance Stage

- Invite the person to go places with you.
- Encourage exercise.
- Offer to listen.
- Reinforce your friendship.
- Encourage rebuilding friendships.
- Offer opportunities for recreation.

Guilt and Anger: The "Why Me?" Stage

Few people experience the loss of someone or something important to them without some feeling of guilt. You tell yourself that you should have done things differently; "if only" is a common thought. You may feel there was more you could have done. Eventually, feelings of guilt will be put in proper perspective.

Anger is also a normal response. Many people feel rage, or at least mild anger. This anger needs to be expressed. However, lashing out at others can cause misunderstandings. Some therapists recommend screaming or yelling in a private place to vent angry feelings without hurting those around you. See page 239 for other ideas.

Adjustment and Acceptance: The "Let's Get On With It" Stage

Life goes on. At some point in the grieving process, you will be better able to come to terms with your loss. Grief will loosen its hold on you, and, in struggling to get on with life, you may discover new opportunities.

Loss teaches us new lessons. You may learn wisdom from your experience and be better able to help others.

Home Treatment

These home treatment guidelines are meant to help when you suffer the loss of a loved one. The same basic principles apply for other losses as well.

- Let yourself cry. If you can let go and just sob, do it.

- Take time to grieve. Actively review mementos, play nostalgic music, and read old letters. Take as much time as you need.

- Talk about your grief. Find a friend who will listen. If your friend tells you to "snap out of it," find a more sympathetic friend.

- Friends may feel awkward about your grief. Let them know that it is all right to talk about the loss. Let them know that they can just talk with you as they did before.

- Get regular exercise. Long walks are particularly healing.

- Eat well.

- Postpone major decisions. Don't be rushed into decisions about moving or changing your job.

- Write your thoughts down in a journal.

- Paint or draw your grief. Find any way possible to express your feelings.

- Join a support group. Contact your local hospital to learn what's available.

Grief - continued

- Talk to your pastor, priest, or rabbi. The clergy can be helpful in understanding and dealing with your loss.

- Books on grieving can help. See Resources N1-2 on page 350.

When to Call a Health Professional

- If you are unable to grieve soon after the loss.

- If you feel furious anger at specific people whom you blame for the loss.

- If social isolation increases after a normal period of mourning. (In some cases, normal mourning can last for years.)

- If there is evidence of self-destructive behaviors (either physical or financial).

- If there are undiminished and overwhelming feelings of guilt.

Memory Loss

Most older adults complain about how their memories work. Many worry that their forgetfulness is an early sign of dementia. Generally, there is no need for concern. Most memory complaints arise from three causes and do not indicate a medical problem.

- With normal aging, it takes more time to retrieve remembered information.

- An ever-increasing amount of information is stored in the memory and more information takes longer to sort through.

- Some people tend to become lax in using their concentration and memory skills. These skills can be relearned.

Most memory complaints are not medically significant. However, the following symptoms could be cause for concern:

- Increasing forgetfulness accompanied by personality changes

- Ignorance about familiar things like the alphabet, numbers, or the names of common objects

- A loss of the ability to remember a short name or phone number long enough to write it down. (This could also be due to a hearing problem.)

Prevention

The best way to prevent memory loss is to stay healthy and actively use your memory. The following guidelines can be particularly helpful:

- Eat well and get plenty of fluids. A balanced low-fat diet, with ample sources of vitamins B6, B12, and folate, will help protect memory.

- Exercise regularly. Exercise helps increase the blood supply to the brain. Your brain needs plenty of oxygen to work properly.

- Minimize the use of medications. Overuse of medications may be the single biggest cause of memory loss among older adults.

- Laugh. Long-term depression has a powerful impact on memory loss and other symptoms of dementia.

- Limit alcohol intake. Alcohol binges affect memory long after sobering up.

- Use it or lose it. The more you use your memory, the longer it will last.

- Develop a positive attitude about your memory. Reject the notion that memory declines with age. If you expect to keep a strong memory, it will be there when you need it. See Resource R1 on page 351.

Home Treatment

- Follow the prevention guidelines above. If you are concerned that memory loss may be due to dementia or Alzheimer's disease, see page 142.

- Deal with reversible causes of memory loss:

The Memory of Meanings

Most of us experience a memory trade-off as we age. What we lose is speed. It takes a little longer to retrieve names, dates, places, and other specific facts. What we gain has been called the "memory of meanings."

As we age we are better able to understand lessons learned from experience. We continually create new linkages between memories. These memory links may slow us down in retrieving facts. However, they are essential in connecting facts so that we understand the meanings behind them. For example, one study has described how younger school teachers remembered more facts about recently reported events, while older teachers better understood what the facts meant.

Another name for the memory of meanings is wisdom. The insight that comes with age and experience is well worth the trade-off in memory speed. Wisdom is a key to understanding people. It is essential too, if we are to help others to improve their lives.

Memory Loss - continued

- Infections can cause significant memory impairment. If you have a fever or other symptoms of an infection, check it out. See page 200.

- Heart disease reduces the flow of blood to the brain and can cause permanent memory loss if left untreated.

- Thyroid, liver, kidney, glucose, and pituitary problems also increase the risk of memory problems.

- Consider hearing or vision problems. If a person does not receive good sensory input, the information will not be well recorded in the memory.

- Get help to deal with depression, if you suspect it is a cause. See page 240.

- Learn new techniques to improve your memory:

  - Take a memory improvement course.

  - Strive to increase attention and concentration. Older people have more difficulty than younger people in dividing their attention between two or more activities. Concentrate on learning new things.

- Keep written notes. Write all your plans on a calendar that you refer to often.

- To keep track of your eyeglasses, buy an eyeglass cord and keep them around your neck.

- To avoid misplacing your keys, keep them in a special place by the door.

- To avoid forgetfulness when cooking, use a timer with a loud bell.

- To remember medications, ask your pharmacist for a medications box with different compartments for each day and time of day.

When to Call a Health Professional

- If you are concerned that memory loss is caused by prescription drugs or specific medical problems.

- If there are severe personality changes, memory problems related to immediate recall, or difficulty in remembering familiar things like the alphabet.

Sleep Problems

Insomnia can mean any of three problems:

- Trouble getting to sleep (more than 45 minutes)

- Frequent wakenings (six or more times a night)

- Early morning awakening

However, none of these are real problems unless they cause you to feel chronically tired. If you are less sleepy at night or wake up early, but still feel rested and alert, there is little need to worry.

Short-term insomnia, lasting from a few nights to a few weeks, is usually caused by worry over a stressful situation. Long-term insomnia, which can last months or even years, is most often caused by general anxiety, medications, chronic pain, depression, apnea (breathing problems), or other physical disorders.

Prevention

- Get regular exercise but avoid strenuous exercise within two hours before bedtime.

- Avoid alcohol, caffeine, and smoking before bedtime.

- Avoid drinking more than a glass of fluid before bedtime.

Sleep Apnea

Apnea is a common problem that causes people to stop breathing for at least 10 seconds at a time during sleep. It is particularly common in older, overweight men. People with apnea complain of extreme daytime sleepiness in spite of seeming to sleep at night.

Apnea usually occurs when the pharynx muscles in the throat become too relaxed during sleep. The relaxed muscles cause the pharynx to collapse and obstruct the airway. After a moment, the low level of oxygen causes an automatic response that triggers breathing to start again.

- Find out if you stop breathing for 10 or more seconds while you sleep.

- Lose weight.

- Sleep on your side. Attach a sock with a tennis ball in it to the back of your pajama top. This will keep you from rolling onto your back.

- Practice the six steps for better sleep on page 252.

- Avoid sleeping pills and alcohol.

- If surgery is proposed, ask for a second opinion.

Sleep Problems - continued

Home Treatment

- Don't take sleeping pills. They can cause daytime confusion, memory loss, and dizziness. Continued use of sleeping pills actually increases sleeplessness in many people. Instead, get regular exercise and drink a glass of warm milk before bedtime. Try the following six-step formula for two weeks:

1. Save your bed for sleeping. Don't eat, watch TV, or even read in it.

2. Save your sleep for bedtime. Don't take naps. (However, naps are fine if you don't have sleep problems.)

3. Forget "bedtime." Go to bed only when you feel sleepy.

4. Get out of bed and leave the room any time you lie awake for more than 15 minutes.

5. Repeat steps 3 and 4 until it is time to get up.

6. Get up at the same time each day, no matter how sleepy you are.

- Review all of your prescription and over-the-counter medications with a pharmacist to rule out drug-induced sleeplessness.

- Read about anxiety on page 239.

When to Call a Health Professional

- If you suspect medication side effects are causing sleep problems.

- If a month of self-care doesn't solve the problem.

Suicide

When people get depressed, they sometimes think of suicide. This is particularly true of older adults facing retirement or major illness. Depression is the most common cause of suicide. Fortunately, depression is treatable. Occasional thoughts of suicide are not a problem. However, if they recur often and linger, they should be treated seriously.

Home Treatment

These guidelines will help you help someone else.

- Use your common sense and a direct communication approach to determine if the risk of suicide is great.

  - Does the person feel there is no way out of the crisis?

  - Has the person developed a suicide plan?

  - How does the person plan to do it?

  - When does the person plan to do it?

- Who else has the person told?

- Speak as matter-of-factly as possible and show concern but not undue anxiety.

- Show understanding and acceptance of the person. Help the person to think through the crisis and what caused it.

- Arrange for yourself or another trusted person to stay with the person for that day or night to show concern and offer support.

When To Call A Health Professional

- If a person indicates that preparations have been made for the suicide.

- If you have questions or doubts about how great the risks are. Look in the telephone book under Suicide Prevention to find a local hot-line number.

Withdrawal

Withdrawal is the continuous desire to avoid other people. Withdrawal can be a passive person's attempt to make others feel responsible for him. Withdrawn people tend to stay in their rooms, talk less than they used to, and avoid group activities.

There are three basic reasons for withdrawal: depression, low-self-

esteem, and shyness. Fear can also cause a person to withdraw.

Home Treatment

- A withdrawn person is suffering from a breakdown in communication. Be very patient in letting them talk with you. It may require long periods of silence.

- Provide continued support and caring even if it is not recognized.

When to Call a Health Professional

- See Seeking Professional Help on page 235.

Even if you are on the right track,
you will get run over if you just sit there.
Will Rogers

19

Fitness

"Step right up, ladies and gentlemen, and get your wonder wellness pills. When taken as directed, just one pill a day will make the lame walk, the weak strong, and the tired full of energy.

"Just one pill a day, taken as directed, will put that special sparkle back in your eyes. It will make your body look better, your mind work faster, and your memory last longer.

"Just one pill a day, taken as directed, will protect you against arthritis, heart disease, high blood pressure, obesity, diabetes, osteoporosis, and even cancer. Step right up and get your wonder wellness pills today."

While wonder wellness pills don't really exist, the claims made above can be achieved. The "wonder" is not in the pills, but in the directions on how to take them--for wonder wellness pills to work, they must be taken daily after 30 to 60 minutes of exercise or moderate activity.

The Benefits of Exercise

No amount of exercise can guarantee a long life. However, even moderate amounts of exercise can improve the likelihood of a healthy life. Along with a positive attitude and a healthy diet, your fitness level plays a major role in how well you feel, what illnesses you avoid, and how much you enjoy life.

But what if you've never exercised before? Can you still benefit? You bet! Even if you have avoided all exertion for the past 50, 60, or 70 years, you can gain from improved fitness. That's absolutely guaranteed! How fit you were as a child, a youth, a young adult, or last year, doesn't count for much. What matters is how consistent you will be today, tomorrow, and in the years to come.

Consistency is the most important, the most basic, and the most often neglected part of fitness. Consistency in regular exercise or moderate

Benefits of Exercise - continued

activity delivers all of the fitness benefits.

The benefits of fitness are universal. If you exercise regularly, you can expect to gain all the advantages. You don't have to be friendly, mind your manners, dress correctly, or even vote. You must simply be consistent in your daily exercise. That's all. Really.

If you don't normally exercise, even 10 minutes of walking per day can make a difference. To get most of the benefits of exercise, as listed on page 257, you need to spend only 30 minutes every day walking, swimming, or doing other forms of moderate exercise. When you are consistent, it takes very little to keep the body in tune.

While 30 minutes a day may be enough exercise to keep the doctor away, you may want to try a little more. The benefits of exercise usually increase as your commitment to fitness increases. The optimal duration of exercise is discussed on page 260.

Wonder Wellness Pills

Wonder Wellness Pills are guaranteed to improve your life. If taken as directed, one pill per day will give you 10 amazing benefits. You will:

1. Feel great, refreshed, and alive!
2. Lose unwanted pounds!
3. Become more fit!
4. Sleep more soundly!
5. Meet more friends!
6. Improve your sex life!
7. Fit into your clothes!
8. Be more creative!
9. Be calmer!
10. Go for the gusto!

(First prescribed by Don Ardell)

WONDER WELLNESS PILLS

Directions For Use:
Wonder Wellness Pills must be taken within 24 hours of 60 minutes of moderate exercise.

Benefits of Exercise

For Promoting Health

Improve your self-image. People who remain fit usually feel better about themselves.

Improve your endurance. People who remain fit can walk farther, work harder, and dance longer than those who do not.

Sharpen your thinking. Exercise improves circulation to the brain and overall alertness.

Improve your sleep.

Control your weight.

Regulate your energy level.

Improve your balance and flexibility. Exercise can help you maintain a full range of motion.

Keep your bones strong and healthy.

Improve your appetite.

Protect your joints.

Fitness is fun. You meet interesting people and go interesting places.

For Preventing Illness

Avoid or recover from depression. Exercise is a great way to bounce back from depression, grief, or the blues.

Avoid or recover from heart disease. Exercise reduces your risk of heart attack, stroke, and high blood pressure.

Avoid or recover from dementia. Exercise can help many who have reversible dementia to regain full mental alertness.

Avoid insomnia.

Avoid obesity.

Avoid or control diabetes.

Improve balance and flexibility, which can reduce falls and automobile accidents.

Prevent osteoporosis.

Prevent constipation.

Reduce disability caused by arthritis.

Poor fitness is no fun. You miss many interesting opportunities because you are unable to participate.

Benefits of Exercise - continued

Overall fitness includes a balance of endurance, strength, and flexibility. Whether you are an Olympic athlete, an octogenarian, or both, these three aspects of fitness are important--particularly as you grow older.

Endurance Training: Aerobic Exercise

Endurance is a measure of how well you can handle physical stress and strain. In fitness terms, it is how long you can dance, entertain grandchildren, or garden without feeling tired or exhausted. Training to improve endurance is called aerobic conditioning. It is the most popular form of fitness and the most beneficial. Most of the benefits of fitness come from endurance training.

Aerobic means "with air." Your muscles need oxygen to work. In aerobic conditioning, your muscles are worked slowly enough that they can get all the oxygen they need from your breathing. That's why you should be able to continue aerobic exercises for a long time.

Exercising too fast causes you to become breathless. Continuing to exercise when you are out of breath is called anaerobic (without air) exercise. Anaerobic exercise is hard and stressful, such as running as fast as you can or sprinting up a flight of stairs. Because it makes you breathless, you cannot continue it for long.

Beginning a Fitness Program

For most people, moderate exercise is not a health hazard. However, if you can answer yes to any of the following questions, talk with your doctor before beginning an exercise program.

- Have you been told that you have heart trouble?

- Do you have chest pains?

- Do you often feel faint or dizzy?

- Do you have arthritis or other bone or joint problems that might be aggravated by improper exercise?

- Have you ever had high blood pressure?

- Do you have diabetes? (You may wish to see your doctor to review the effects of increased exercise on your insulin needs.)

- Are you over 60 years, unaccustomed to vigorous exercise, and planning to do more than moderate activity or walking?

- Are there other reasons not mentioned here that raise doubts about the safety of exercise for you?

Aerobic exercise is steady and rhythmic, and can be maintained for a long time without causing breathlessness. For most people, walking is a good aerobic exercise. Studies show that slower and steadier aerobic exercise provides more health benefits than fast and exhausting anaerobic exercise.

The point of aerobic conditioning is to train your body to use more and more oxygen from your breathing. The more efficiently your body uses oxygen, the longer your muscles can work before you become out of breath.

When people start thinking about exercise to increase endurance, three questions generally come up:

1. How hard should I exercise?

2. How often should I exercise?

3. How long should I exercise?

The answers may surprise you.

How Hard Should I Exercise?

Nice and easy does it. Exercise does not have to be intense to be of value. In fact, if you exercise too hard, you get less benefit from the workout than if you go at a moderate pace.

There are two easy ways to monitor how hard you are exercising. One way is to gauge the amount of exertion you feel (the Borg Scale); the other is to check your pulse (target heart rate).

The Borg Scale

The Borg Scale is simple, yet effective. Just ask yourself how difficult the level of exercise seems to you.

Ideally, you would exercise at a level around 13 (Somewhat Hard). If you get above 15 (Hard), slow down. If you have dropped below 11 (Fairly Light), you can safely increase the intensity of your exercise.

Your Target Heart Rate

You can tell if you are exercising too much or too little by taking your pulse during exercise. You can figure out your target heart rate with the help of the chart on page 261.

Try to find an exercise level that keeps your pulse in the target range for your age. If you are just starting an exercise program, gradually work up to a level of exertion that gets your heart rate into the target range. Regular exercise even at that level is

6	7	8	9	10	11	12	13	14	15	16	17	18	19	20
	VERY, VERY LIGHT		VERY LIGHT		FAIRLY LIGHT		SOME-WHAT HARD		HARD		VERY HARD		VERY, VERY HARD	

Borg Scale: Try to keep your exercise around level 13 (Somewhat Hard).
If it goes above 15 (Hard), slow down.

Aerobic Exercise - continued

helpful. However, if you are exercising above your target rate, slow down. You will get more fitness benefits if you stay within the target range.

Important note: The target heart rate method does not work for those with pacemakers or using pulse-altering medications. If you are not sure, ask your physician or pharmacist.

How Often and How Long Should I Exercise?

From a scientific point of view, exercising every day may not be necessary. Most studies show that exercising three times a week is enough to improve fitness. However, many people find that they can be more consistent if they try to exercise every day. When you do something daily, it quickly becomes a habit. In the long run, it will be easier and more effective.

With exercise, harder is not better, but longer is. While people can show marked improvement with as little as ten minutes of exercise per day, extending your exercise time will increase your rewards.

This is true at least up to one hour of exercise per day. Beyond that, there may be diminishing returns and increasing risk of injuries.

Start with a time commitment you can comfortably accomplish, then look toward increasing not the intensity, but the duration of your exercise.

Taking Your Pulse

Your pulse can be felt most easily on the thumb side of your wrist. Place three fingers over the area with only slight pressure. You should feel a rhythmic beating. Count the number of beats you feel for 10 seconds. Multiply this by 6 to get the number of beats for 1 minute.

Example: 13 beats in 10 seconds gives a one minute pulse of 78 (13 x 6 = 78).

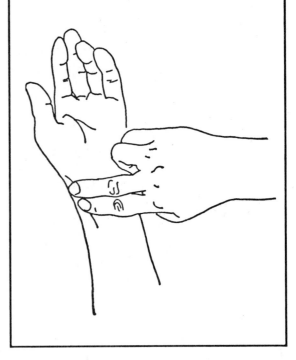

Your Aerobic Style

Aerobic exercise can be as complex or as simple as you like. You can perform a strict series of warm-up exercises, spend a measured amount of time at just the right pulse rate, and follow that with a well-designed sequence of cool-down exercises.

The result will be a constantly improving level of fitness and with it all the benefits of a successful exercise program.

On the other hand, you might regularly spend a comfortable bit of time with your spouse, friend, or neighbor simply walking through the neighborhood, riding a bicycle, gardening, or dancing. Again, the result will be a constantly improving level of fitness and all the benefits of a successful exercise program.

The exercise itself is less important than the regularity of its practice. It matters little whether you swim, walk, mow the lawn, or dance, only that you do it consistently.

Target Heart Rate Range

Age	For 10 Seconds	For 60 Seconds
50	17-23	102-136
52	17-22	100-134
56	16-22	98-131
60	16-22	96-129
64	16-21	94-126
68	15-20	91-122
72	15-20	89-118
76	14-19	86-115
80	14-19	84-112
84	14-18	82-109
88	13-18	79-106
90 and up	13-17	78-104

Try to find an exercise level that keeps your pulse in the target range for your age. Be careful not to exceed the high end of your target heart rate range.

Aerobic Exercise - continued

Walking

Walking is a terrific form of aerobic exercise. It improves endurance, strength, and flexibility. It causes few injuries. It is inexpensive, and enjoyable both alone or with a group.

If you want to start walking for health right now, great. Put the book down and go! It is as easy as that. However, if you like to plan ahead, here are a few things you can do:

- Buy a good pair of walking shoes. They should be comfortable, provide both support and cushion, and not cause blisters.

- Ask around about good places to walk. Most local walkers can give you tips for avoiding traffic, dogs, noise, and other nuisances.

- If there is a shopping mall in your area, ask if there is a morning walking program there. Mall-walking is a very popular way to exercise (and meet new friends) when the weather is bad.

- Take a map. If you don't know the neighborhoods you will walk through, a map can save you a lot of concern about how to get back home.

- If you plan to walk at night, wear reflective clothing and ask about the safest places to walk after dark.

Record Your Progress

When you begin a new exercise program, use a notebook or calendar to record your progress. Each day record:

- What you did

- How long you did it

- How hard your effort was using the Borg Scale on page 259

- Your attitude or motivation for that day

- A record like this will help you measure and improve the most important part of your fitness program: its consistency. As the pages fill up, your record will become an important reminder of how successful you have been in improving your health.

Sample Fitness Journal Walking Program

Date/What	Borg Scale/ Comment
9/1 - 20 min. walk with Mary	14-Felt great
9/2 - 15 min. walk to park	12-Walked very slowly
9/3 - 20 min. walk with Mary	15-Too fast
9/4 - 5 min. walk to store	13-Short, but nice
9/5 - 15 min. to and from Ann's house	13-Beautiful day

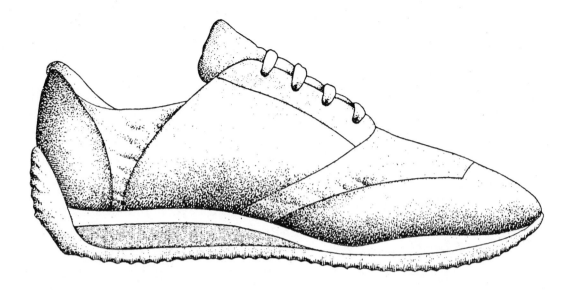

- Just head out from your house at a moderate pace until you start to feel just a little fatigued, and then head back.

- Don't worry about your pace or duration when you're beginning. Consistency is important. As time goes by and your fitness improves, you'll likely find yourself walking longer and picking up the pace.

- Remember these walking tips:

  - Hold your head erect, back straight, and abdomen flat.

  - Point your toes straight ahead.

  - Let your arms swing loosely by your sides.

  - Land on your heel and roll forward to push off the ball of your foot.

- Take long easy strides, but don't strain.

- Lean forward slightly when walking up hills.

- Move at a steady clip, brisk enough to make your pulse and breathing increase, but not so fast that you can't talk comfortably. See the talk/sing test on page 264.

- When you finish, record it in a notebook. See "Record your Progress" on page 262. You will be amazed at how quickly the miles add up.

Aerobic Dance
If you like music and dancing, give aerobic dance a try. It has become a popular form of exercise for both men and women.

Aerobic Exercise - continued

How well you like aerobic dance may depend a lot on the instructor. If the intensity is too high or the music not to your taste, look for another group. The best way to judge both the instructor and the class is to observe the class and the participants before you sign up.

Ballroom dancing and folk dancing offer less strenuous, but very enjoyable and healthful alternatives. If you used to like to dance, try to recapture the spirit.

Swimming

Swimming, water aerobics, and water jogging are forms of aerobic exercise that are particularly kind to your joints and muscles.

Check into what's available in your community. Organized classes are often available, as well as open pool times when you can exercise by yourself.

Biking

Bicycling is another aerobic activity that is kind to joints and muscles. If you are not inclined to head out on the open road (helmet firmly on your head), try a stationary bike. The health benefits are the same even if the scenery doesn't change.

Muscle Strength

As people grow older, they tend to lose muscle. Many think that this muscle loss is strictly due to aging.

The Talk/Sing Test

While you are walking, try the talk/sing test. Like the Borg Scale and the target heart rate, it's a good way to tell if you are going too fast.

The test is simple:

- If you can't talk and walk at the same time, you are going too fast.

- If you can talk and walk, you are doing fine.

- If you can sing and walk at the same time, it would be safe to walk a little faster.

Your exercise is most effective when you're able to talk, but not to sing.

Warm Up and Cool Down

For the first five minutes of your exercise routine, start out slowly and easily so your muscles have a chance to warm up. Try slow walking with gentle arm swings. The key is to do something light.

When you want to end your exercise, be sure to cool down. Gradually slowing your pace and adding some light stretches at the end of the routine will lower your heart rate, improve flexibility, and reduce the chance of stiffness and injury. Try the stretching exercises starting on page 266.

Although age-related hormone changes play a role in muscle loss, that's only a part of the story.

Much more important is the advice: "Use it or lose it." Muscles become soft, flabby, and weak if they are not being used. Muscles that get regular use stay strong.

Muscle strength is important to overall health:

- Strong muscles around joints reduce arthritis pain.

- Strong ankle muscles reduce the chance of sprains.

- Strong abdominal and lower back muscles reduce the chance of back pain.

- Strong arm, shoulder, and leg muscles protect against falls.

Keep your muscles strong to look good, feel good, and do the things that you enjoy doing.

Yoga, tai chi, aerobic dance, walking, swimming, and almost every other form of exercise also include some muscle strengthening. A complete set of flexibility and muscle strengthening exercises can be found on pages 266-275.

Flexibility

A major physical complaint that many older people have is stiffness. Legs, back, neck, and shoulders all seem so much stiffer than before. Is this part of growing older? Maybe not.

Arthritis, with its pain and swelling, reduces joint mobility. However, if you want to be more flexible to avoid injuries, garden more comfortably, walk more smoothly, or get out of bed more easily, you can. Only minutes per day of slow, pleasant, relaxing stretching will give you results you can feel immediately. Stretching after exercise, when your muscles are warmed up, is particularly helpful.

There are many classes that teach stretching and expand your range of motion. Yoga and tai chi classes are particularly good. Swimming will help improve flexibility, and so will the following exercises.

Exercises for Muscle Strength and Flexibility

- Do these exercises slowly.

- Stretch and flex just to the point of muscle tension. Don't overdo it. If it hurts, stop!

- Breathe deeply and don't hold your breath.

- Don't bounce! Bouncing can cause injury.

- For exercises that are particularly helpful for strengthening back and abdominal muscles, see pages 36-39.

Chair Exercises

For neck flexibility:

1. Slow Neck Stretches

- Gently lower right ear toward right shoulder. Hold for 5 counts.

- Bring head back to center.

- Gently lower chin to chest. Hold for 5 counts.

- Lower left ear toward left shoulder. Hold for 5 counts.

- Return to center.

- 5 repetitions.

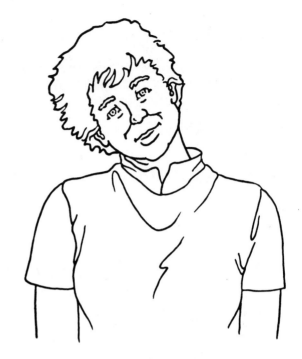

1. Slow Neck Stretches

2. Half-Circles

- Keep chin level.

- Gently turn head to the right. (Try to look over your shoulder.) Hold for 2 counts.

- Gently turn head to the left. Hold for 2 counts.

- 5 repetitions.

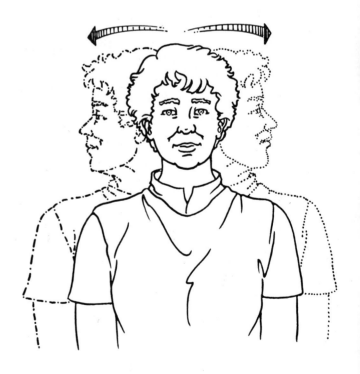

2. Half-Circles

For shoulder flexibility:

3. Shoulder Rolls

- Keep arms relaxed and at your sides.

- Trace large circles in the air with your shoulders.

- Roll forward 5 times, backward 5 times.

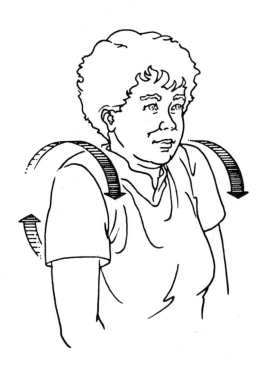

3. Shoulder Rolls

For hand and wrist flexibility:

4. Finger Squeezes

- Extend arms in front at shoulder level, palms down.

- Slowly squeeze fingers to form a fist, then release. 5 repetitions.

- Turn palms up. Squeeze and release. 5 repetitions.

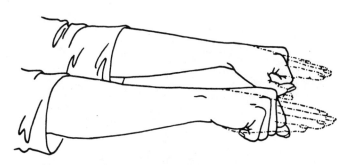

4. Finger Squeezes

5. Hand Circles

- Extend arms in front at shoulder level. Keep elbows straight, but not locked.

- Rotate wrists in small circles.

- 10 circles to the left, 10 to the right.

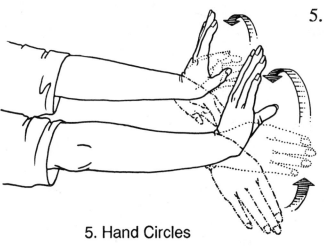

5. Hand Circles

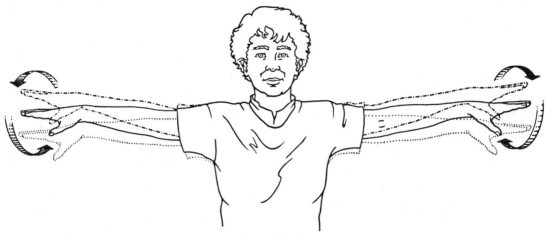

6. Arm Circles

To strengthen shoulders and upper back:

6. Arm Circles

- Raise arms at sides to shoulder level. Keep elbows straight.

- Rotate arms from shoulders in small circles.

- 10 circles forward, 10 backward.

For trunk flexibility:

7. Spine Twists

- Sit or stand with back straight, head high.

- Raise arms out to sides at shoulder level. Bend elbows upright, palms facing forward.

- Keep hips and knees facing forward.

- Slowly twist your upper body to the right. Hold for 5 counts.

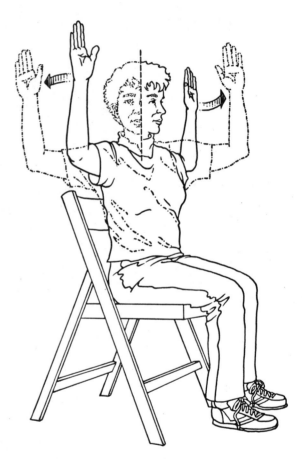

7. Spine Twists

- Return to center, then twist to the left. Hold for 5 counts. 5 repetitions.

To strengthen knee flexors and lower abdomen:

8.   Knee Lift

- Raise right knee to chest or as far upward as possible. Do not pull up with hands.

- Return to starting position.

- Bring left knee to chest.

- 5 repetitions for each leg.

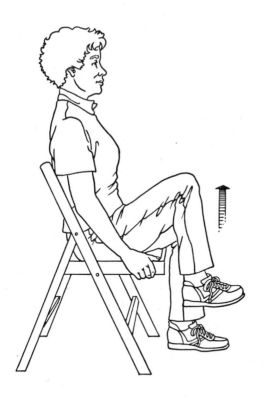

8. Knee Lift

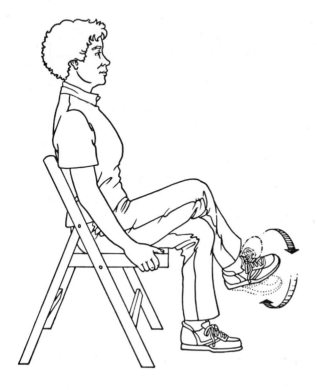

For ankle flexibility:

9.   Ankle and Foot Circling

- Cross right leg over left knee.

- Slowly rotate right foot, making large circles.

- For each ankle, 10 rotations to the right, 10 to the left.

9. Ankle and Foot Circling

Stretch Tubing Exercises

For these exercises, you will need a 24-inch length of surgical latex tubing with knots tied at each end. Some exercise "stretchies" are sold commercially at fitness stores.

When you use a "stretchie," go slowly and be careful not to overstretch.

At the start, hold each stretch for a count of 5. You may increase the time as you get stronger. Keep a firm grip, too. You don't want it snapping back at you!

For arm and shoulder flexibility and strengthening and for chest and back strengthening:

10. Stretch and Reach

- Shorten the stretchie by holding one end and the middle of the tube.

- Raise both arms overhead, hands facing forward.

- Reach for the ceiling with alternate hands.

- 5 repetitions each hand.

11. Overhead Stretch

- Raise both arms overhead, hands facing forward.

- Tighten tubing by slowly pulling both arms away from center. Do not overstretch.

- 5 repetitions.

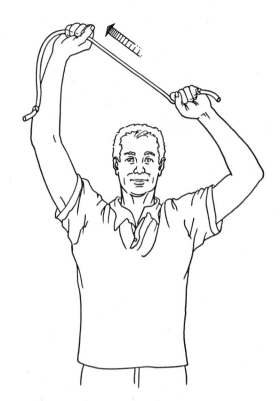

10. Stretch and Reach

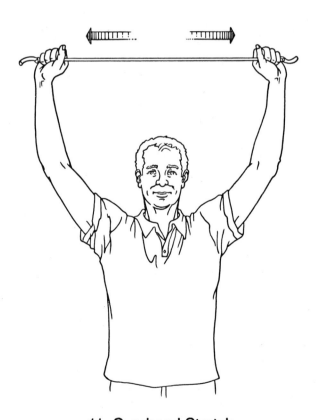

11. Overhead Stretch

12. Up-down Stretch

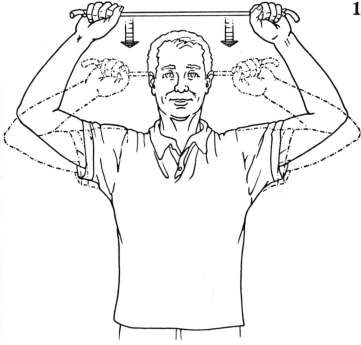

- Raise both arms overhead.

- Stretch the tubing slightly.

- Bend elbows and lower arms, bring tubing to rest on shoulders behind the head.

- 5 repetitions.

12. Up-down Stretch

13. Chest-level/Lap-level Stretch

- Raise arms out in front to shoulder level.

- Pull hands apart, stretching tubing.

- 5 repetitions.

- Drop arms to the level of your lap.

- Pull hands and arms away from your body to the sides.

- 5 repetitions.

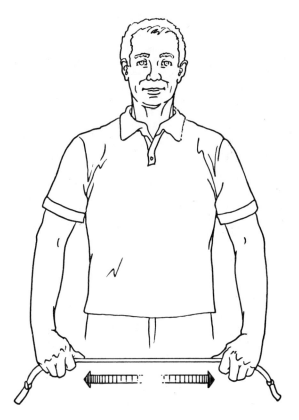

13. Lap-level Stretch

Exercises Done While Standing

Hold onto a sturdy object, like the back of a chair, for these exercises.

For upper torso flexibility:
14. Side Stretch

- Hold onto chair back with right hand.

- Stand with feet shoulder-width apart.

- Bring left arm up and over your head. Slowly bend over to the right. Feel the stretch in your left side. Hold for a count of 10.

- Slowly return to an upright position. 5 repetitions for each side.

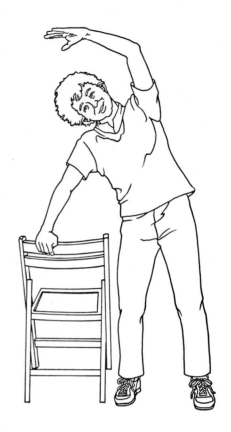

14. Side Stretch

For stretching calf muscles:
15. Leg Stretch

- Face the back of the chair and point toes straight ahead.

- Stretch right leg out behind you. Keep left leg slightly bent.

- Press your right heel to the floor. (You should feel a pull in your right calf muscle.)

- If you cannot get your heel down, move your legs closer together. Hold for a count of 5.

- Repeat 5 times for each leg.

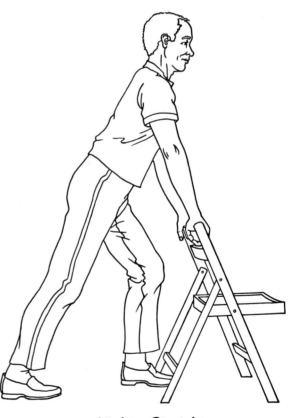

15. Leg Stretch

To tone and strengthen legs and ankles:

16. Heel Raises

- Hold onto chair back.

- Rise up on toes. Hold for 5 counts.

- Repeat 10 times.

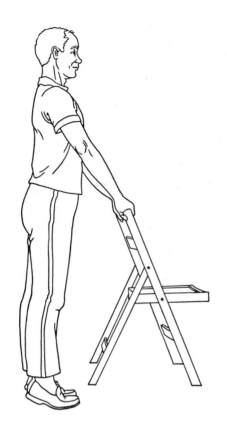

16. Heel Raises

For balance and hip flexibility:

17. Leg Swings

- Stand up straight with your left side to the chair back. Hold on with your left hand.

- Gently swing your right leg to and fro. Repeat 10 times.

- Repeat 10 times with your left leg.

- Use controlled movements. Don't let your body move to the back or front when you swing your leg.

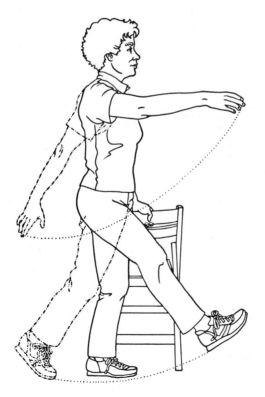

17. Leg Swings

Floor Exercises

To stretch lower back and hamstrings:

18. Knee-to-Chest Leg Lifts

- Lay on back.

- Bring knee to chest.

- Lift leg up.

- Hold for 5 counts.

- Bring knee back to chest.

- Repeat 5 times with each leg.

To strengthen stomach and neck muscles:

19. Head and Shoulder Curl

- Lie on your back with your knees slightly bent.

- Keep arms at sides.

- Curl head and shoulders off floor. Hold for 5 counts.

- Return to starting position.

- Repeat 10 times.

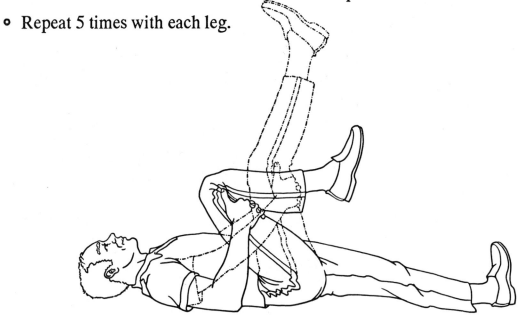

18. Knee-to-Chest Leg Lifts

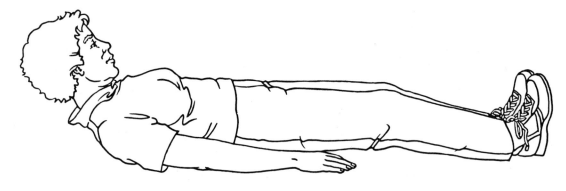

19. Head and Shoulder Curl

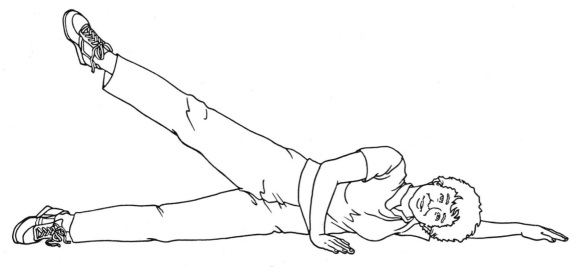

20. Side-lying Leg Lifts

To strengthen and tone hip and thigh muscles:

20. Side-lying Leg Lifts

- Lie on left side, legs extended.

- Raise right leg as high as is comfortable.

- Lower to starting position.

- Repeat 10 times for each leg.

Setting Your Fitness Goals

Are you as strong, flexible, and physically fit as you would like to be? If you are, wonderful. We hope this chapter has helped you to re-affirm the exercise that you are already doing. However, if you would like to make some improvements, here's one piece of advice: try to improve only a little bit at a time.

You can walk a mile only by taking one step at a time. You can become a lot better at something only by becoming a little better lots of times.

Consistency always brings success. Each success may be only a small one, but small triumphs can quickly add up to something that will make a big difference in your life.

Use the assessment on the next page to help you reach your long-term fitness goals. Begin by taking one small step at a time.

Fitness Assessment

Step 1: Where are you now?

On the scales below, a "10" is the highest fitness level that you could possibly obtain if you spent all of your time on these components. A "1" on the scale is no activity at all.

For each component, circle your current level of fitness.

Fitness Component

Endurance Training: 1 2 3 4 5 6 7 8 9 10
             No activity   Very active

Muscle Strength: 1 2 3 4 5 6 7 8 9 10
             Very weak   Very strong

Flexibility: 1 2 3 4 5 6 7 8 9 10
             Very stiff   Very flexible

Step 2: How fit would you someday like to be?

For each component, circle the level of fitness that you would like to reach.

Step 3: Pick one area for improvement.

Put a "*" next to the fitness component that you want to improve first. Describe your long-term goal here:

_____

_____

_____

Step 4: Set your one-month goal.

For the fitness area that you picked, what can you do to move your fitness up only one point on the scale? Pick a one-month goal that you think you can accomplish with easy but consistent effort. Write your short-term goal here:

_____

_____

_____

Step 5: Keep up the good work.

When you have reached your one-month goal, pick a new one. Each new goal can be an extension of the old one, or a small step toward improving another fitness component. Good luck and happy fitness.

Eat less sugar,
Eat less fat,
Beans and grains,
Are where it's at.
Unknown

20

Nutrition

As you age, three things happen that change both what you need to eat and what you choose to eat.

- Your body slows down. As your metabolic rate decreases, you need less energy from food.

- Physical changes may make different foods more attractive to you. For example, soft foods may become more appealing to those who have dental problems. Sweet or salty foods appeal to those whose sense of taste and smell has changed. Also, a reduced ability to sense thirst may cause you to drink less.

- Your lifestyle may change. You may eat alone more or have less motivation to prepare complete meals.

Compare your body to an automobile, which needs both gasoline and oil to run well. The calories in your food are your body's gasoline; you must burn calories to make your body go. The vitamins, minerals, and fiber in your food are also essential. Like regular oil changes, these nutrients keep the body in balance and running smoothly.

As you age, you get better mileage-- that is, you need fewer calories. However, you still need the same number of oil changes. Overall, you need less food but the same amount of nutrients. Eating healthy foods becomes even more important as you get older.

Nutritional Guidelines

Good nutrition can be as simple or as complex as you want. On the simple level, everything you need to know is covered in the following seven guidelines. For a more complete view of nutrition, read the entire chapter.

Nutritional Guidelines - cont'd

Seven Simple Guidelines for Good Nutrition

1. Eat a variety of foods. Include a daily selection of:

    - Fruits

    - Vegetables

    - Whole-grain and enriched breads, cereals, and grain products

    - Milk, cheese, and yogurt

    - Meats, poultry, fish, eggs

    - Legumes (dried peas and beans)

2. Maintain a healthy weight. See Weight Control on page 295.

3. Choose a diet low in fat, saturated fat, and cholesterol. Fats have twice as many calories per ounce as any other food. See page 285.

4. Choose a diet with plenty of vegetables, fruits, and grain products. Complex carbohydrates pack the most nutrients per calorie. See page 280.

5. Use sugars only in moderation. Sugars have no vitamins, minerals, or fiber. See page 282.

6. Use salt and sodium only in moderation. For some people, sodium increases blood pressure. See page 293. If you are

not salt-sensitive, sodium may not be a problem for you.

7. Drink alcohol only in moderation. Alcohol is high in calories and has no nutrients.

The 80-20 Rule

If you eat good, nutritious foods 80 percent of the time, you can relax the remaining 20 percent and eat what you like.

If most of your food is wholesome, an occasional ice cream cone, order of fries, or double-decker cheeseburger won't hurt you. On the other hand, if most of the food you eat is high in fat, sugar, and salt, a few "health foods" and vitamin pills are probably not going to improve your health.

Good eating should become a regular habit, but it need not make you abandon other foods you like. "All things in moderation" is the key.

Good Nutrition: A Basic Plan

Eat a variety of foods from these six basic food groups. Eat more from the breads and cereals, fruits, and vegetables groups than from the other groups.

Most people who follow this plan will get all the vitamins, minerals, and other nutrients that their bodies need and have little trouble controlling their weight.

Good Nutrition: A Basic Plan

Breads/ Cereals/ Starches	6-11 servings/day	Breads and cereals make up the foundation of the plan. High in carbohydrates and low in fat, whole grains are a good choice. A serving size is 1 slice of bread, 1/2 to 3/4 cup of cooked cereal, pasta, or rice, or one ounce of ready-to-eat cereal.
Vegetables	3-5 servings/day	Fresh or fresh-frozen vegetables are best. Eat a variety of vegetables for a balanced diet.
Fruits	2-4 servings/day	Use fresh or fresh-frozen fruits. Variety is important. A serving is about 1/2 cup.
Milk/Milk Products	2-3 servings/day	Drink two cups per day of low-fat milk or eat two servings per day of other dairy products, such as low-fat yogurt or cheese.
Meat/Meat Alternatives	2-3 servings/day	Choose low-fat meats, poultry, or fish. Avoid high-fat meats. One serving of cooked meat is two to three ounces. Beans, seeds, and other high-protein foods can be substituted for meat.
Fats/Oils/ Sweets	Use sparingly	Fats and oils increase the risk of heart disease and cancer. See page 285 to reduce the amount of fat you eat. To reduce the number of empty calories you get from sugar, see page 284.

Breads, Cereals, and Starches

Contrary to popular belief, bread, potatoes, rice, and pasta are not fattening! These starchy foods are actually good for you.

Starches are carbohydrates. Carbohydrates have only half the calories per ounce that fat has. Starches also contain large amounts of vitamins, minerals, fiber, and water.

Starchy foods become fattening only when you add fat to them. Try substituting non-fat yogurt or salsa for butter and sour cream on baked potatoes. Use fresh vegetable and tomato sauces instead of rich cream sauces on pasta.

Fruits and Vegetables

Fresh fruits and vegetables are good for you. They are high in carbohydrates and contain vitamins, minerals, and fiber. Most people think they taste good, too.

Fruits and vegetables are most nutritious when they are eaten fresh and raw. The longer they are cooked, frozen, or canned, the fewer nutrients remain. Even so, cooked or canned vegetables are better than none at all, and fresh-frozen vegetables may have more nutrients than "fresh" vegetables that have been left in the refrigerator for several days.

When you do cook vegetables, steam them lightly rather than cooking directly in water to retain more vitamins.

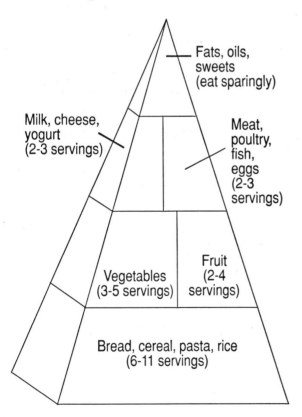

The Eating Right Pyramid
(USDA)

Fats, oils, sweets (eat sparingly)

Milk, cheese, yogurt (2-3 servings)

Meat, poultry, fish, eggs (2-3 servings)

Vegetables (3-5 servings)

Fruit (2-4 servings)

Bread, cereal, pasta, rice (6-11 servings)

Better Nutrition Can Be Easy

You don't have to change your whole diet at once. Just pick one improvement and stick with it:

- Buy only whole-grain bread.
- Buy only skim or low-fat milk.
- Use less oil for cooking and buy vegetable oil that is liquid at room temperature.
- Eat fish at least twice a week.
- Drink an extra glass of water when you wake each morning.

Vegetables Against Cancer

Vegetables are important for good basic nutrition. They also have been shown to protect against cancer.

A diet rich in a wide variety of vegetables can cut the risk of stomach, colon, and lung cancer.

Cruciferous vegetables, such as cabbage, cauliflower, broccoli, brussels sprouts, and kohlrabi appear to reduce the risk of breast, stomach, and colon cancers.

Vegetables and fruits high in vitamin A (such as spinach, carrots, tomatoes, apricots, and cantaloupe) and vitamin C (all citrus fruits, broccoli, green and red peppers) also provide some protection against cancer.

How many servings of fruits and vegetables do you need? Nutritionists recommend three to five servings of vegetables and two to four servings of fruit every day. One-half to one cup of cooked or raw vegetables provides one serving. A small apple and a half-cup of fruit juice or canned fruit each provide one serving.

Fiber

Fiber has no vitamins or nutrients, yet it is important to health.

Fiber helps to digest food and excrete waste. Together with fluids, fiber prevents constipation. A lack of fiber increases risks for colon and bowel cancer, constipation, and diverticulosis.

Fiber provides "bulk" for your diet. It stimulates the colon to keep waste moving out of the bowels. Without fiber, waste moves too slowly, increasing the risks of illness.

Do you need more fiber? If your bowel movements are large, soft, and easy to pass, you are probably getting plenty of fiber. If they are small, hard, and difficult to pass, more fiber and water may help. See page 99 for more information on constipation.

There are lots of ways to increase the amount of fiber in your diet. Wheat bran helps make stools soft and prevents constipation, but it is better to get fiber from many sources than to just add a tablespoon of bran to your cereal every morning. The fiber in fruit, legumes, and oats helps lower cholesterol. The fiber from legumes lowers both cholesterol and blood glucose.

To increase fiber in your diet:

- Eat at least five servings of fresh fruits and vegetables a day. Raw or lightly steamed fruits and vegetables contain more usable fiber. Much of the fiber is in the skins. Wash well before eating.

Fiber - continued

- Use whole-grain products such as brown rice (instead of white rice), whole-wheat spaghetti, whole-wheat tortillas, and whole-grain cereals.

- One slice of whole-grain bread per meal adds much needed fiber. The first ingredient listed should say "whole-wheat flour." If it just says "wheat flour," it means white flour, from which much of the fiber has been removed.

- Eat more cooked dried beans, peas, and lentils. These high-fiber, high-protein foods can replace some of the high-fat, no-fiber meats in your diet.

- Eat fruits with edible seeds: kiwis, figs, blueberries, and raspberries.

- Eat more of the stems of broccoli and asparagus.

- Popcorn is a good high-fiber snack. However, be aware of added oil, butter, and salt. Use an air popper to eliminate oil, and flavor with salt substitute or herb mixtures.

Water

Water is a nutrient that is particularly important as we age. One easy way to improve your diet is to drink a big glass of water when you first get up each morning. Active people need six to eight 8-ounce glasses (two quarts) of water a day. If you drink other fluids, you can get by with less, but plain water is best. (For those of you who need the calcium, don't forget to keep up your milk intake, too.)

If you are concerned about overloading your bladder, follow these tips:

- Drink most of your water in the morning and early afternoon.

- Increase your water intake gradually by a glass per week to give your body a chance to adjust.

Sugar

What's wrong with sugar? It comes from a vegetable (sugar beets or sugar cane), is relatively cheap, tastes good, is fat-free, and is even a carbohydrate. How can sugar be all that bad?

From a health point of view, the biggest problem with sugar is that it is stripped of all vitamins, minerals, and fiber. What is left are crystals of pure calories.

Coffee

There is no convincing evidence that a moderate amount of caffeine (two to three cups of coffee per day) will do you any harm if you are healthy.

Caffeine is mildly addictive. Abrupt reductions in caffeine intake may cause headaches. Gradual reductions in caffeine work well.

Magic Elixir Promises Health Benefits!

Ladies and gentlemen, the miraculous magic elixir pictured here is essential to your continued good health. Not only does it taste great, but this magic tonic is guaranteed to protect your health in seven important ways.

1. Aids Digestion! Helps to unlock the nutrients in your food.

2. Prevents Constipation! At last, regularity is within your grasp.

3. Aids Circulation! Builds up the volume of your blood.

4. Helps Protect against Colds, Coughs, Flu, and Sore Throats! You will stay healthier than ever before.

5. Prevents Urinary Tract Infections! You will be "in the clear" and avoid troublesome irritations.

6. Protects You from the Heat of the Sun! Helps cool your body to guard against heat stroke.

7. Helps Weight Loss! Controls your appetite with no adverse side effects.

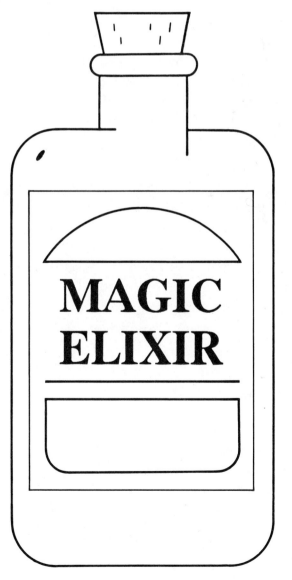

Yes, ladies and gentlemen, this miracle tonic is available today. It is one hundred percent natural and totally calorie-free. There are no artificial flavorings or preservatives whatsoever. Best of all, it can be delivered fresh to your home for less than a penny a day!

Drink one glass more today than you did yesterday, and two more than that tomorrow...until you are hooked on eight or more glasses a day. Order yours today by contacting your kitchen faucet, your Perrier dealer, or a mountain spring.

Yes, you guessed it right...the magic elixir is WATER!

Sugar - continued

In moderation, sugar does little harm. However, if too many of your calories come from sugar, you will either gain too much weight or get too little of the other nutrients you need.

A little sugar now and then hardly makes a difference; a teaspoon has only 16 calories. Unfortunately, the average American gets about 16 percent of total calories from sugars. The national dietary guidelines suggest that no more than 10 percent of calories should come from sugar.

How much sugar you eat is a question of balance. If you are happy with your weight, eat a good balanced diet, and brush and floss your teeth daily, you need not worry. However, if you think that your sweet tooth is adding too much to your weight, try the following:

- Beware of hidden sugars in many processed foods. Flavored yogurt, breakfast cereals, and canned goods often have sugar added. Check the label for words that end with "-ose," like dextrose, fructose, sucrose, lactose, and maltose. All are sugars. Corn syrup is another common form of sugar.

- Be aware that you lose tastebuds as you age. Foods need more sugar to taste as sweet as they used to. However, if you cut back on sugars, your taste will adjust.

Artificial Sweeteners

If you try to trick your sweet tooth by using artificial sweeteners, don't overdo it. Questions remain unanswered about the long-term safety of large doses of both saccharine and aspartame (Nutrasweet).

Although artificial sweeteners do help you avoid high-calorie sugars in the short run, their use does not increase success in weight-loss diets. Weight-loss success is much more dependent upon reducing calories from fat.

- You can reduce the sugar in baked goods by up to one-half without affecting the texture.

- When you do have very sweet desserts, take a small serving and eat it with very small bites. It will give you the same pleasure, but with fewer calories. Desserts like Jello, hard candy, and fruit ices contain lots of sugar, but little or no fat. Desserts like ice cream, cakes, cookies, and sweet rolls usually contain lots of sugar and lots of fat. Sugar-only desserts are much less a problem than high-fat desserts.

- The best way to cut back on sugar is to eat other carbohydrates. They are more nutritious and tend to fill you up.

- Remember that all sugars are basically alike. Honey, brown or raw sugar, and corn syrup have no significant advantage over other sugars.

Fats in Foods

Fat--the butter, lard, cream, oil, and grease in foods--accounts for 37 percent of the calories in the average American diet. Fat is appropriately named because it is more than twice as fattening per gram as carbohydrates or protein.

How much fat is too much? The U.S. Dietary Guidelines recommend that less than 30 percent of total calories be from fat. Certainly, changing from a diet that contains 37 percent fat to one that contains 30 percent fat will slow the development of heart disease, reduce cancer risk, and

---

Calculating Percent Fat

Each gram of fat is 9 calories. To calculate the percent of calories that are fat, multiply the grams of fat times 9 and then divide by the total number of calories.

For example, an 8 ounce serving of 2% milk has 5 grams of fat and 130 total calories.

$$\frac{5 \text{ grams fat} \times 9 \text{ calories/gram}}{130 \text{ calories}}$$

$$= 35\% \text{ calories from fat}$$

---

improve your overall diet. But is it enough?

Many nutritionists suggest a 30 percent fat diet is still too much for a healthy diet. A 20 percent fat diet will slow heart disease even more. There is now good evidence that a 10 percent fat diet can even reverse the buildup of plaque in the arteries. However, a 10 percent fat diet is not easy to maintain. Based on your other heart disease risks, you may wish to set a goal for how much fat to include in your diet. A nutritionist can help you with a menu plan to meet your goal.

All fats, in excess, cause problems, but some fats are more troublesome than others. The table on page 286 describes four basic types of fat. If heart disease is a concern, cut back on saturated and hydrogenated fats. Both saturated and polyunsaturated fats increase risks for breast cancer.

16 Simple Ways to Reduce Fat in Your Diet

When eating meat:

1. Choose lean cuts of meat, such as tenderloin, flank steak, chuck, top and bottom round, or lean veal. Use more poultry and fish

2. Remove all visible fat before cooking.

3. Remove skin from poultry before cooking.

4. Broil or bake instead of frying.

Fats - continued

5. Reduce serving sizes and don't eat seconds.

6. Replace some meat proteins with vegetable proteins. See page 290.

When using dairy products:

7. Use low-fat or skim milk.

8. Choose low-fat cheeses: gruyere, Jarlsburg swiss, mozzarella, ricotta, parmesan, or any cheese made from part-skim milk. Avoid or limit whole-milk cheeses (Swiss and cheddar).

Types of Fat			
Type	**Characteristics**	**Examples**	**Effect on Body**
Saturated Fats	Solid at room temperature. Most animal fats, especially red meats.	Butter, cheese, sour cream, cream, lard, lamb, beef, coconut oil, palm oil, cocoa butter, cream	Increases risk of heart disease and stroke. Raises cholesterol in blood.
Monounsaturated Fats	Liquid at room temperature. Will partially harden in the refrigerator.	Avocados, peanut oil, olive oil, some fat from fish and chicken, most nuts	Lowers LDL ("bad") cholesterol. May reduce risk of heart disease and stroke.
Polyunsaturated Fats	Liquid, even when refrigerated.	Corn, soybean, sunflower seed, safflower, walnut, canola, and cottonseed oils	Lowers total cholesterol levels in blood. May reduce risk of heart disease and stroke.
Hydrogenated Fats	Polyunsaturated fat that has been hardened artificially and converted to saturated fat. Solid at room temperature.	Shortening, peanut butter, and margarine are made from oils that are hydrogenated. Check the labels on crackers and "vegetable" oils.	Possible adverse effect on heart and hormonal systems. Raises cholesterol in blood.

9. Substitute low-fat cottage cheese and yogurt for cream, sour cream, cream sauce, and cream soup.

In cooking:

10. Saute vegetables with one tablespoon of oil or less. Add a little water if needed. Also try cooking with other liquids, such as wine, defatted broths, or cooking sherry.

11. Add oil to a pre-heated pan. Less goes further this way.

12. Flavor vegetables with herbs and spices instead of butter and sauces.

13. Experiment with using less oil than is called for in recipes. You may need to increase other liquids.

In general:

14. Avoid crackers, chips, non-dairy creamers, and margarines with hydrogenated oil, palm oil, coconut oil, or cocoa butter.

15. Eat plenty of carbohydrates to fill you up (fruits, vegetables, grains, bread, pasta, etc.).

16. Let salads go naked or modestly clothed in lemon juice.

Cholesterol

Cholesterol is a waxy fat that is both produced by the human body and found in animal products. Some cholesterol is needed for every cell to function. Unfortunately, excess cholesterol builds up as deposits inside the arteries. Cholesterol deposits are the major cause of heart attacks and strokes.

Along with how much you smoke, how high your blood pressure is, and your family medical history, the amount of cholesterol in your blood is a good predictor of your risk for heart disease and stroke. The more cholesterol you have, the higher the risk. However, not all cholesterol is bad.

Good Cholesterol

Fat is carried in your blood attached to protein. The combination is called a lipoprotein. Two lipoproteins are the main carriers of cholesterol: low-density lipoprotein and high-density lipoprotein.

Low-density lipoprotein (LDL) acts like a fat delivery truck. It picks up cholesterol from digesting food and delivers it to the cells. When more cholesterol is ready for delivery than the cells can take, the delivery truck drops off the extra cholesterol on the walls of the arteries. A lot of LDL cholesterol in your blood increases your risk of heart disease and stroke.

The other type of cholesterol, high-density lipoprotein (HDL), works like a garbage truck. It picks up excess cholesterol from the walls of the arteries and takes it to the liver. A lot of HDL cholesterol decreases your risk of heart attack and stroke.

Cholesterol - continued

Cholesterol Testing

Basic cholesterol tests are easy, quick, and inexpensive. They do not require fasting for accurate results. If your total cholesterol is over 200 mg/dl (milligrams per deciliter), have it checked annually.

Otherwise, a test every five years is appropriate. Call your local health department to learn if free or low-cost cholesterol tests are available.

Special cholesterol blood tests can measure the amounts of both low-density and high-density lipoprotein in your blood. These tests do require fasting for accurate results. The charts on page 289 describe how cholesterol levels are related to risks.

How to Reduce Your Cholesterol

- Eat less total fat. Because your body makes cholesterol from fat, just cutting back on cholesterol in food is not enough. You must cut back on fats in foods as well. Follow the guidelines for eating less fat on page 285.

- Buy a cooking oil that is liquid at room temperature and use less of it. See the table on page 286.

- Eat more fish. Most fish contain Omega-3 fatty acids that help to lower blood cholesterol and triglycerides. In general, fish with darker flesh such as mackerel, lake trout, herring, fresh albacore tuna, sturgeon, whitefish, salmon, and halibut have more Omega-3 oils. Two to three servings of fish per week are sufficient. The safety and value of fish oil supplements is not yet fully known.

- Exercise more. Exercise increases your protective HDL cholesterol level.

- Quit smoking. Quitting can increase your HDL levels.

- Lose extra pounds. Dropping back to your ideal weight can increase HDL levels and lower your total cholesterol.

- Eat more fiber from oat bran, cooked dried beans, dried peas, lentils, and fruits with pectin (apples). These foods contain a high amount of soluble fiber, which lowers overall cholesterol.

- Consult with a registered dietitian. A nutritionist can help you lower your fat consumption to 30 percent, 20 percent, or less of total calories, based on your goal. A consultation is a good idea if your total cholesterol level is over 200. Nutritional counseling is very important if the level is over 239.

Medication for High Cholesterol

Several drugs are effective in lowering cholesterol. However, they have side effects and require lifelong use. Unless LDL levels are very high, most physicians require six months

Total Cholesterol Guidelines - mg/dl total cholesterol

under 180	under 200	200 - 239	over 240
Most desirable	Low risk. No changes required	Moderate risk. Re-test yearly. Eat a low-fat diet.*	High risk. Re-test yearly. Check LDL levels. Eat a low-fat diet.*

LDL Cholesterol Guidelines

LDL Level (mg/dl)	Heart Disease Risk Level	Action *
Under 130	Desirable	No action required. Recheck in 5 to 10 years.
130 - 159 (no other risks)	Moderate	Low-fat diet. Recheck in 5 years.
130-159 (with other risk factors)	High	Very low-fat diet. Recheck in 4 weeks and annually.
Over 160 (no other risk factors)	High	Very low-fat diet.Recheck in 4 weeks and annually.
Over 160 (with other risk factors)	Dangerous	Very low-fat diet. Recheck in 1 week. Consider medications.
Over 190	Dangerous	Very low-fat diet. Recheck in 1 week.Consider medications.

* Low-fat diet: less than 30 percent of calories from fat; less than 10 percent from saturated fat; no more than 300 mg of cholesterol per day

Very low-fat diet: less than 20 percent of calories from fat; less than 7 percent from saturated fat; no more than 200 mg of cholesterol per day

Cholesterol - continued

of diet changes before prescribing drugs. Medications may be prescribed sooner if the person has diabetes, hypertension, or other conditions that increase the risk of heart attack or stroke.

Protein

Protein is important for maintaining healthy muscles, tendons, skin, bones, blood, hair, and internal organs. The need for protein does not decrease with age. Fortunately, most older adults have no problem getting all the protein they need. (Most Americans eat twice the required amount of protein.)

While protein deficiencies are rare, they do occur. If you don't drink milk and eat little meat because of problems with chewing, you would be smart to track the amount of protein you are eating.

Complete Or Incomplete Protein?

Proteins are made up of different combinations of 22 amino acids. The absence of any one of these can cause problems. Your body manufactures 13 of the necessary 22. The remaining nine must come from what you eat. Animal sources of protein (milk, eggs, meat, and fish) have all nine in the proportions that your body requires.

Although vegetables are also high in protein, no single vegetable has all

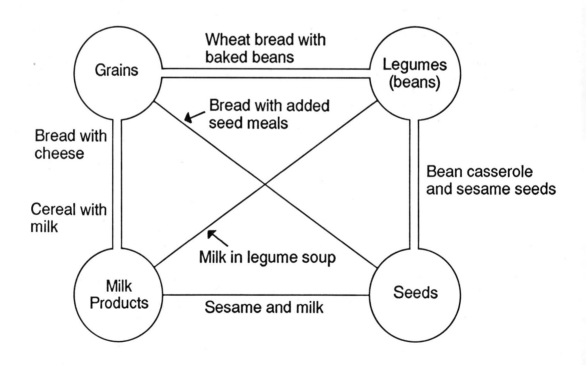

Protein Complement Chart
If you eat foods from two groups connected by a
double line, you get a complete protein.

How to Calculate Your Protein Needs

You can calculate your protein requirements by multiplying your weight in pounds by 0.36 grams. For example, if you weigh 150 pounds, you would need 54 grams per day of protein (150 x .36 = 54). You can get that from the recommended daily servings of basic foods:

Protein	Grams
Bread/ cereal: 4 servings	12 grams
Fruit: 2 servings	0 grams
Vegetables: 2 servings	4 grams
Milk: 2 servings	16 grams
Meat: 2 servings	28 grams
Total	**60 grams**

---

nine essential amino acids in the right proportions. Fortunately, it is possible to obtain all nine by combining vegetables with other foods. The Protein Complement Chart on page 290 shows how foods can complement each other's protein.

Vitamins

Vitamins are exciting! These tiny, unseen elements of food have no calories, yet are essential to good health. There are 13 known and necessary vitamins.

Four vitamins (A, D, E, and K) are fat-soluble and can be stored in the liver or in fat tissue for a relatively long time.

The other nine are water-soluble and can be retained by the body only for short periods. They include:

- Thiamine
- Riboflavin
- Niacin
- Pantothenic acid
- Biotin
- Folate
- Vitamin B6
- Vitamin B12
- Vitamin C

Vitamin Deficiencies

For most people, a well-balanced diet of fresh food provides all the vitamins needed for good health. Your best protection against vitamin deficiency is to eat at least two servings of fruit and three servings of vegetables every day.

Vitamin deficiencies are somewhat more common in older adults because they tend to eat less food. If you are eating less than 1500 calories per day, you may wish to consider a low-dose vitamin/mineral supplement.

Vitamins - continued

Vitamin Buyer's Guide

It remains unproven whether vitamin and mineral supplements significantly improve health. However, if you choose to take vitamins, the following guidelines may be helpful.

- Choose a balanced, multiple-vitamin/mineral supplement rather than one containing a specific vitamin or mineral, unless it has been medically prescribed. Too much of any one mineral can interfere with the body's ability to use other minerals.

- Choose a supplement that provides nearly one hundred percent of the RDA (Recommended Dietary Allowance) for vitamins and minerals in about equal proportions.

- Avoid taking much more than 100 percent of the RDA for any vitamin. This is particularly important for the fat-soluble vitamins A, D, E, and K. Because these vitamins are stored in the body, large doses can build up to toxic levels.

- Vitamins lose potency over time. Look at the expiration date before you buy.

- There is no chemical difference between brands of vitamins. High-priced vitamins sold door-to-door are no different than those you can get from the grocery store.

Minerals

Minerals in food help regulate the body's water balance, hormones, enzymes, vitamins, and fluids. The various minerals must be maintained in delicate balance to ensure proper functioning of the systems they serve. Eating a good variety of fresh foods is the best way to get all of the minerals you need.

To date, 60 minerals have been discovered in the body. Twenty-two are known to be essential to health. The three that we know most about are calcium, iron, and sodium. All three are particularly important to older adults.

Calcium

Calcium is the primary mineral needed for strong bones. However, calcium cannot be used in the bones without vitamin D. The human body can make its own vitamin D if exposed to direct sunshine. Otherwise, vitamin D can be obtained through fortified milk, fish, and egg yolks.

Women lose calcium from their bones more rapidly after menopause. Calcium in the diet combined with exercise and vitamin D can help slow the loss of bone mass. This prevents or postpones osteoporosis and the brittle bone fractures that it causes. See page 50 for more on osteoporosis.

A total of 1500 milligrams of calcium per day is recommended for post-menopausal women. If you like milk, getting enough calcium is not a big problem. A quart of skim milk has about 1100 milligrams. Non-fat yogurt is another good source.

While dietary calcium is preferred, low-dose calcium supplements may also help to slow bone loss. One 500 milligram TUMS (calcium carbonate) tablet provides about 200 milligrams of calcium. If you are unable to bring the calcium in your diet up to 1500 milligrams per day, one TUMS tablet per day may help. However, don't use supplements to justify not drinking milk.

You can easily overdo calcium supplements. Too much calcium can actually decrease bone strength. Calcium and phosphorus are needed in a one-to-one balance for good bone health. If too much calcium is added, the imbalance causes problems.

Sodium

Most people get far more sodium than they need. Our bodies need only 500 milligrams of sodium per day. However, the average American eats five to ten times that amount. Anything over 2500 milligrams of sodium per day is probably too much.

For people who are sodium-sensitive, excess sodium is a direct cause of high blood pressure. About ten percent of people under age 40 are sodium-sensitive. However, sodium sensitivity increases with age. People over age 50 are less able to excrete excess sodium. The older you are,

---

Milk or Lactose Intolerance

People whose bodies produce too little of the enzyme lactase have trouble digesting the lactose sugar in milk. In some people, lactose intolerance increases with age. Symptoms include gas, bloating, cramps, and diarrhea.

Tips for dealing with lactose intolerance include:

- Eat small amounts of dairy products at any one time.

- Drink milk only with snacks or meals. The other foods slow down digestion time, giving your enzymes more time to digest the milk.

- Cheeses usually do not cause symptoms. Most of the lactose is removed during processing.

- Yogurts made with active cultures provide their own enzymes and cause fewer tolerance problems.

- Pre-treated milk, enzyme treatments, and enzyme tablets are available. Ask your pharmacist.

- Severe lactose intolerance may increase your need for calcium supplements. Ask your physician.

---

the more likely it is that an excess of sodium will increase your blood pressure.

Sodium - continued

Salt is the most familiar form of sodium. About 40 percent of salt is pure sodium. If all of your sodium came from salt, one-quarter teaspoon per day would be all that you needed. However, sodium also comes hidden in foods that don't taste at all salty. Two ounces of cheddar cheese, for example, have over 400 milligrams of sodium. Sodium is also a major ingredient of monosodium glutamate (MSG), disodium phosphate, and baking powder.

If you want to cut back on the sodium in your diet:

- Shift your focus from cheese to milk. A cup of 1 percent milk has more protein and calcium than an ounce of cheddar cheese, but fewer calories, less fat, and 20 percent less sodium.

- Eat lots of fresh or frozen fruits and vegetables. These foods have very little sodium.

- Beware of "convenience" foods. Ready-mixed sauces and seasonings, frozen dinners, canned or dehydrated soups, and salad dressings are usually packed with sodium. Read the label before deciding if the convenience is worth it.

- Don't put the salt shaker on the table, or get a shaker that allows very little salt to come out.

Creative Salt Substitute

Mix together and put in a shaker:

1/2 teaspoon cayenne pepper

1/2 teaspoon garlic powder

1 teaspoon each:

    basil

    black pepper

    mace

    marjoram

    onion powder

    parsley

    sage

    savory

    thyme

- Always measure the salt in recipes and use half of what is called for.

Iron

Small amounts of iron are needed to make hemoglobin, which carries oxygen in the blood. Most older adults need about 10 milligrams of iron per day. People who have increased blood loss from ulcers or who regularly take aspirin, anticoagulants, or arthritis medications may need more. An inexpensive blood test can determine if you need additional iron.

For more iron in your blood:

- Drink a glass of orange or other citrus juice along with eating a bowl of iron-enriched cereal.

Vitamin C helps you absorb more iron from food.

- Increase absorption of vegetable iron by eating meat, poultry, or fish along with the vegetables. The iron in animal tissues (heme iron) is more easily absorbed than the iron in vegetables.

- Cook in cast-iron pots to increase the iron content of foods.

- Avoid tea. It interferes with iron absorption.

Iron-deficiency Anemia

Iron-deficiency anemia in older adults is usually caused by chronic blood loss from the digestive tract (via ulcers, colon cancer, or long-term daily use of aspirin). Chronic blood loss of any kind depletes the body's store of iron. Symptoms of iron-deficiency anemia include paleness and fatigue. A blood test is needed to confirm the diagnosis. Because anemia can be caused by many things other than an iron deficiency, medical attention will be needed.

Iron Supplements

Older adults who eat fewer than 1500 calories per day may wish to consider an iron supplement. However, too much iron can cause a number of serious medical problems. A low-dose ferrous-form iron supplement of no more than 20 milligrams per day is safe for most people. Do not take more without consulting your physician. Take the supplement with citrus juice.

Weight Control

People come in all shapes and sizes. Weight control can help you stay the shape and size that you want to be.

Focus on Fat, Not Weight

For health and looks, fat control is more important than weight control. Too much body fat increases your risk of diabetes, heart disease, and stroke. Ideally, body fat is around 15 percent of total weight for men and about 22 percent for women. A fitness or nutritional counselor can measure your body fat percentage. Check with your local YMCA.

Exercise Makes it Easier

Regular exercise will raise your metabolism, the rate at which your body burns calories. Your body continues to burn more calories long after you stop exercising. Regular exercise increases your metabolic rate. Exercise makes it much easier to lose weight and, more importantly, body fat.

Exercise Keeps You Strong

If you diet without exercising, you will lose both fat and lean muscle mass. As a result, you may feel weak and stop the diet. However, if you exercise regularly while you are losing weight, you will tend to lose mostly fat and very little lean muscle mass.

Never Go Hungry

You may think that skipping a meal is a good way to lose weight. It is not. Going hungry, even for a few hours, will cause your metabolic rate

Weight Control - continued

to drop. You will gain more weight if you eat a single 1800-calorie meal each day than if you eat three 600-calorie meals. In fact, you can eat up to 20 percent more calories and maintain your weight if those calories are spread throughout the day.

Fat Foods Make You Fat

Cutting down on the fat in your diet is guaranteed to have a positive effect on your overall body fat. If you shift from a 2000-calorie diet that is 40 percent fat, to a 2000-calorie diet that is only 30 percent fat, your body fat will go down. If you drop to a 20 to 25 percent fat diet, you can lose even more. You will see a substantial weight loss without any loss of energy. See the ways to reduce fat in your diet on page 285.

Get Help From Your Friends

The food customs and habits of friends and family affect what you eat. Ask those you spend time with to help you succeed with your weight-control plan. Specifically, ask friends and family to:

- Celebrate events with nutritious foods.

- Make water and low-calorie snacks available.

- Serve low-calorie options with meals.

- Offer small servings.

Help Yourself to Good Thoughts

Develop a positive attitude about yourself. Think of yourself as healthy, take pride in making good nutrition choices, and have confidence that you can control your weight.

We don't stop playing because we grow old,
we grow old because we stop playing.
Anonymous

21
Stress and Relaxation

Stress is the physical, mental, and emotional reactions you experience as the result of changes and demands in your life.

Stress is part and parcel of common life events, both large and small. It comes with all of life's daily hassles, traffic jams, long lines, petty arguments, and other relatively small irritations. Stress also comes with crises and life-changing events-- events that may seem to gang up on you in later life:

- Illness or disability

- Children leaving home

- Loss of job or retirement

- Marriage difficulties or divorce

- Loss of a spouse

- Grandparenthood

- Caregiving responsibilities

All of these events may force you to adjust, whether you are ready or not. Unless you can regularly unlock and release tension that comes with stress, it can greatly increase your risks for physical and mental illness.

Because many major life events are beyond your power to control, take charge of those aspects of your life that you can manage. One major change doesn't mean that all areas of your life must change. Continue to participate in the same activities you did before the event happened.

Not all stress is bad. Positive stress, or eustress, is a motivator, challenging you to act in creative and resourceful ways. When changes and demands overwhelm you, then distress, or negative stress, sets in. This chapter has specific techniques that you can use to cope with stress in your life and to help you feel your best.

What Stress Does to the Body

The immediate physical reaction to stress is universal:

- Heart rate increases to move blood to the muscles and brain.

- Breathing rate increases.

- Digestion slows.

- Perspiration increases.

- Pupils dilate.

- You feel a rush of strength.

- Blood pressure increases.

Chemicals released by the pituitary and adrenal glands automatically trigger these physical reactions at the first sign of alarm. Your body is tense, revved-up, and ready for action. For primitive humans, these reactions held an advantage in the face of sudden danger. They allowed for better survival by either "fight-or-flight." Today, however, it is not so acceptable to either fight or run away from your stressors (although we often wish we could).

After the natural "alarm" reaction to a real or perceived threat, our bodies stay on alert until we feel that the danger has passed. When the stressor is gone, the brain signals an "all clear" sign to the pituitary and adrenal glands. They stop producing the chemicals that caused the physical reaction; the body then returns to normal.

Problems with stress occur when the brain fails to give the "all clear" signal. If you stay in the alarm state too long, you begin to suffer from the consequences of constant stress. Unrelieved stress can lead to many health problems.

The Symptoms of Negative Stress

Distress can affect your body, your emotions, and your behavior. Everyone responds to stress differently.

Distress and Illness

Chronic negative stress often plays a role in the following health problems:

- Accidents
- Arthritis
- Asthma
- Cancer
- Colds
- Colitis
- Diabetes
- Fatigue
- Headaches
- Heart disease
- High blood pressure
- Insomnia
- Muscle aches
- Sexual dysfunction
- Ulcers

Physical Signs

- Muscle tension

- Headaches

- Chest pain

- Upset stomach

- Diarrhea or constipation

- High blood pressure

- Racing heartbeat

- Cold clammy hands

- Fatigue

- Profuse sweating

- Rashes

- Rapid, shallow breathing

- Shaking, tics, jumpiness

- Poor or excessive appetite

- Weakness, exhaustion, lethargy

- Dizziness

Emotional Signs

- Anger

- Low self-esteem

- Depression

- Apathy

- Irritability

- Fear and phobic responses

- Difficulty concentrating

- Guilt or worry

- Agitation, anxiety, panic

Behavioral Signs

- Alcohol abuse

- Drug abuse (includes medications)

- Increase in smoking

- Disrupted sleep

- Overeating

- Memory loss

- Confusion

Some people seek to relieve their distress by smoking, drinking, overeating, or taking pills. There is a better way. Spare your body the dangerous side effects of tobacco, alcohol, and tranquilizers by learning to control your stress levels. You can do this by using your body to soothe your mind and by using your mind to relax your body.

You can relieve stress by taking simple steps to relax your body. Three excellent ways to do this are by deep breathing, muscle relaxation, and physical exercise.

Breathing

Breathing is the key to life and to good mental and physical health. Our bodies need air to nourish vital organs and purify blood. Even though we have been taking in air since the moment of birth, proper breathing is a skill that many of us have to

Breathing - continued

relearn. All too often, we breathe in short, incomplete breaths which leave stagnant air in the lungs and reduce the flow of oxygen to the blood.

The way we breathe is also a sign of stress levels. Breath-holding and hyperventilation (the feeling of not being able to catch your breath) are symptoms of nervous tension. Whenever you find yourself doing either, use it as a cue to take time out to relax. The following deep-breathing exercises will promote good health and bring on relaxation.

Roll Breathing

The object of roll breathing is to develop full use of your lungs. It can be practiced in any position, but is best learned lying on your back, with your knees bent.

1. Place your left hand on your abdomen and your right hand on your chest. Notice how your hands move as you breathe in and out.

The Benefits of Deep Breathing

- Reduces stress
- Oxygenates mind and body
- Purifies blood
- Warms cold hands and feet
- Nourishes vital organs

---

2. Practice filling your lower lungs by breathing so your left hand goes up and down while your right hand remains still. Always inhale through your nose and exhale through your mouth.

3. When you have filled and emptied your lower lungs 8 to 10 times with ease, add the second step to your breathing. Inhale first into your lower lungs as before but then continue inhaling into your upper chest. As you do so, your right hand will rise and your left hand will fall a little as your stomach draws in.

4. As you slowly exhale through your mouth, make a quiet, whooshing sound as first your left hand and then your right hand falls. As you exhale, feel the tension leaving your body as you become more and more relaxed.

5. Practice breathing in and out in this manner for three to five minutes. Notice that the movement of your abdomen and chest is like the rolling motion of waves rising and falling.

Practice roll breathing daily for several weeks until you can do it almost anywhere. It becomes an instant relaxation tool anytime you need one.

Caution: Some people get dizzy the first few times they try roll breathing. Get up slowly and with support.

The Relaxing Sigh

During the day you may catch your-self sighing or yawning. This is generally a sign that you are not get-ting enough oxygen. Sighing and yawning are the body's ways of remedying the situation. A sigh releases a bit of tension.

1. Sit or stand up straight.

2. Sigh deeply, letting out a sound of deep relief as the air rushes out of your lungs.

3. Don't think about inhaling--just let the air come in naturally.

4. At the end of each out-breath, shake your hands away from your body as a symbol that you are throwing your tension away.

5. Repeat this procedure 8 to 12 times whenever you feel the need for it. Experience the feel-ing of relaxation.

Massage for Head, Neck, and Shoulders

Massage is nature's remedy for headaches, and for tight shoulders, neck, and back. It is best to have someone do the massage for you. However, many of the following steps (2, 5, 6, 7) can be done on your own.

1. Have your partner sit comfort-ably upright in a chair with feet flat on the floor. Stand behind her.

2. Using both hands, gently mas-sage across the top of the shoulders with a kneading motion.

3. Apply gentle but firm and even pressure with your thumbs across the top of the shoulders. Work your way toward the neck and then back across to the ends of the shoulders.

4. Locate the vertebrae at the base of the neck. Place your thumbs on either side of the vertebrae and apply gentle but firm pres-sure away from the spine. Con-tinue down the back. Do **not** press on the spine itself.

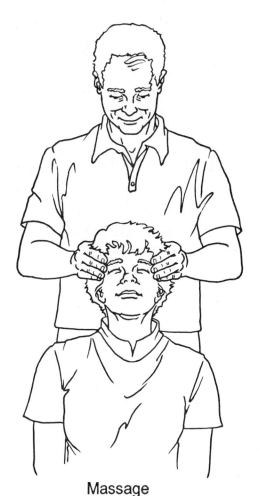

Massage

Massage - continued

5. Locate the indentations at the base of the skull on either side of the spine at the back of the head. Apply gentle rotating pressure with your thumbs.

6. Use three fingers on each hand to massage the jaw muscles. Have your partner clench her jaw. You will easily find the muscles that need to be rubbed. Make sure your partner's jaw is unclenched before you massage the muscles.

7. Gently massage the temples using your fingertips. Work across the forehead and back to the temples.

8. Bring your hands back to the shoulders and allow your hands to say "goodbye" with a few soft calming strokes.

Progressive Muscle Relaxation

In response to stressful thoughts or situations, the body reacts with muscle tension. Deep muscle relaxation can calm the mind as well as ease muscle tension.

Procedure and Muscle Groups

Choose a place that is dimly lit and where you will be undisturbed. Pick a seating arrangement that will support your body. Beds, couches, cushions, and recliner chairs are all good.

You can use a pre-recorded tape to help you go through all the muscle groups or you can do it by just tensing and relaxing each muscle group in the manner described below.

Tense each muscle group for 4 to 10 seconds (hard, but not to the point of cramping), then give yourself 10 to 20 seconds to release and relax. Tense:

1. **Hands** by clenching them.

2. **Wrists and forearms** by extending them and bending the hands back at the wrist.

3. **Biceps and upper arms** by clenching your hands into fists, bending your arms at the elbows, and by flexing your biceps.

4. **Shoulders** by shrugging them.

5. **Forehead** by wrinkling it into a deep frown.

6. **Eyes and bridge of nose** by closing the eyes as tightly as possible.

7. **Cheeks and jaw** by grinning from ear to ear.

8. **Around the mouth** by pressing the lips together tightly.

9. **Back of the neck** by pressing the head back hard.

10. **Front of the neck** by touching the chin to the chest.

11. **Chest** by taking a deep breath and holding it, then exhaling.

12 **Back** by arching the back up and away from the supporting surface.

13. **Stomach** by tightening it into a tense knot.

14. **Hips and buttocks** by pressing the buttocks together tightly.

15. **Thighs** by clenching them hard.

16. **Lower legs** by pointing the toes back toward the face and then pointing the toes away from the face.

Exercise: The Natural Way to Relax

Try walking, swimming, dancing, biking, and stretching your way to relaxation. A regular fitness program is a natural way to change stress into relaxation. Exercise strengthens the body's ability to meet sudden stressful demands, lowering susceptibility to both mental and physical illness.

Vigorous exercise also stimulates the body's production of endorphins. These chemical messengers from the brain produce feelings of euphoria. Exercise will help you tap into your brain's own natural tranquilizers.

Mental Relaxation

Much of the stress that we experience is generated by worried thoughts or by negative "self-talk." By learning to quiet your mind, you can calm and relax your body.

You will need a stretch of uninterrupted time and a quiet place for all the following mind-relaxing techniques.

Relaxation Response

The relaxation response is the exact opposite of a stress response. It slows the heart rate and breathing, decreases blood pressure, and helps relieve muscle tension.

Technique
Adapted from Herbert Benson, M.D.

1. Sit quietly in a comfortable position with eyes closed.

2. Begin progressive muscle relaxation. See page 302.

3. Become aware of your breathing. As you exhale, say the word "one" silently or aloud. Concentrate on breathing from your abdomen and not your chest.

4. Continue this for 10 to 20 minutes. As distracting thoughts enter your mind, don't dwell on them, just allow them to drift away.

5. Sit quietly for several minutes, until you are ready to open your eyes.

6. Notice the difference in your breathing and your pulse rate.

Don't worry whether you are successful in becoming deeply relaxed. The

Relaxation Response - cont'd

key to this exercise is to remain passive, to let distracting thoughts slip away like waves on the beach.

Practice one or two times a day for 10 to 20 minutes, but not within two hours after a meal. When you have set up a routine, the relaxation response should come with little effort.

Imagery

Imagery is a relaxation skill that requires some imagination. In your mind's eye, create a mental picture of a relaxing scene, such as basking in warm sun or strolling through a beautiful garden. Let yourself experience the peace of your mental scene. Your body will respond with lowered pulse rate, controlled breathing, and muscle relaxation.

1. Begin with your choice of a physical relaxation technique (progressive muscle relaxation, stretching, deep breathing.)

2. Use the relaxation response to calm your mind and focus your attention. Then, vividly create, within your mind, the picture of a peaceful scene. It can be a sunny beach, or a mountain meadow, whatever works for you. Concentrate on the sights, sounds, and smells of your special place, letting the tranquility of the setting permeate your being. Stay as long as you like.

3. Continuing with your deep breathing, slowly come back to reality. Remember, this is your special place to relax. Come here any time you wish.

Color Imagery

1. Close your eyes and scan your body for any points of tension. Associate the color red with this tension.

2. Take a deep breath and change the color from red to blue. Let all the tension go. Experience the relaxation associated with the color blue.

3. Imagine the color blue becoming darker and darker. Relax further with each deepening shade.

4. Practice changing from red to blue with each daily hassle you confront. Use the color blue as your cue to relax.

Eye Relaxation (Palming)

1. Put your palms over your closed eyes. Block out all light without putting too much pressure on your eyelids.

2. Visualize the color black. You may see other colors or images, but focus on black.

3. Continue with this for two to three minutes, thinking and focusing on black. Slowly open your eyes, gradually getting accustomed to the light. Feel the relaxation in the muscles around your eyes.

A person of sixty can grow as much as a child of six.
Gay Gaer Luce

22

Mental Wellness

Health is more than just the absence of illness, it is a measure of well-being. In addition to physical health, our mental and spiritual wellness account for much of our quality of life.

Mental wellness is what we think and feel about ourselves. While this chapter does not discuss any particular illness or health problem, it may do more for your health than any other. The ideas presented in the next few pages are both simple and profound. If you learn how to put them to use, they can boost your health and vitality in immeasurable ways.

The Mind-Body Connection

You have heard of psychosomatic illness--when a person "thinks" himself into being sick. Evidence now supports the idea of psychosomatic "wellness." For sickness and for health, what you think has at least some influence on you.

Medical science is making remarkable discoveries about how expectations, emotions, and thoughts affect health. This science is called "psychoneuroimmunology" or PNI. It studies how the brain communicates with the rest of the body by sending chemical messengers into the blood.

Researchers have found that one function of the brain is to secrete substances that can help you to better health. Your brain can create natural painkillers, called endorphins, gammaglobulin for fortifying your immune system, and interferon for combatting infections, viruses, and even cancer.

Your brain can combine these and other substances into a vast number of tailor-made prescriptions for what ails you. The substances that your brain produces depend, in part, on your thoughts and feelings.

Mind-Body Connection - cont'd

Your immune system's ability to heal is linked to your state of mind. Your level of optimism and your expectations of what could happen can affect what goes on inside your body.

Positive Thinking

People with positive attitudes generally enjoy life more. Aside from that, are they any healthier? The answer is often yes.

Optimism is a resource for healing. Optimists are more likely to overcome pain and adversity in their efforts to improve their outcomes. For example, optimistic coronary bypass patients generally recover more quickly and have fewer post-operative complications than people who are less hopeful.

Conversely, pessimism seems to aggravate ill health. One long-term study showed that people who were pessimistic in college have significantly higher rates of illness through age 60.

People seem to develop a tendency toward either optimism or pessimism at an early age. However, even if your general outlook on life tends to be gloomy, you can enjoy psychosomatic wellness by using your brain to support your immune system.

The Hardy Personality

Some people have more basic protection from disease than others. Their immune systems appear to be naturally more efficient. Researchers studying these people have identified three factors in their personalities that stand out.

1. Hardy people show a strong commitment to self, work, family, and other values.

2. Hardy people have a sense of control over their lives.

3. Hardy people generally see change in their lives as a challenge rather than as a threat.

Boosting Your Immune System

Your body's immune system responds to your thoughts, emotions, and actions. In addition to staying fit, eating right, and managing stress, the following three strategies will help your immune system function well:

1. Create positive expectations for health and healing.

2. Open yourself to humor, friendship, and love.

3. Appeal to the Spirit.

1. Create positive expectations for health and healing.

Mental and emotional expectations influence medical outcomes. The effectiveness of any medical treatment depends in part on how useful you expect it to be.

The placebo effect is proof that expectations affect health. A placebo is a drug or treatment that provides no medical benefit except for the patient's belief that it will help. On the average, 35 percent of patients

---

Positive Affirmations

An affirmation is a phrase or sentence that sends strong, positive statements to you about yourself. Affirmations can raise both conscious and subconscious expectations about your future. They allow you to improve the reality you create for yourself.

An affirmation can be any positive statement. It can be put in very general terms: "I am a capable person." Affirmations can also be used to help you with a specific problem: "My memory serves me well."

To create an affirmation:

- Express the statement in positive terms. Instead of "My joints hurt less today," say "My joints are strong and flexible."

- Keep it simple and put it in the present. Instead of saying, "I am going to be more relaxed," say "I am completely and deeply relaxed."

- Phrase affirmations with "I" or "my." Try "I am a supportive husband," rather than "Mary appreciates the help I provide."

To practice your affirmation:

- Write it down 10 to 20 times. Then read and reread what you wrote.

- Repeat your affirmation silently or aloud at any time during the day (after waking, during housework, while walking, just before bed, etc.) Repeat it slowly and with conviction.

- If negative self-talk comes up, develop affirmations to counteract these contrary thoughts.

- Affirmations help build a more optimistic attitude. However, they are not meant to contradict your true feelings. For problems with depression, anger, anxiety, and other emotional concerns, see Chapter 18.

Immune System - continued

who receive placebos report satisfactory relief from their medical problem, even though they received no actual medication.

While hoping for the best does not ensure success, it can help. Positive expectations are behind much of the success of faith healing and many folk remedies. Negative expectations account for the damage done by voodoo curses. By shifting your expectations from negative to positive, you may bolster your immune system. Here's how:

- Stop all negative self-talk. Restrict any statements that do not promote your recovery.

- Write your illness a letter. Tell it that you don't need it anymore and that your immune system is now ready to finish it off.

- Send yourself a steady stream of affirmations. See page 307.

- Visualize health and healing. See Visualization on this page.

- Become a cheerleader for your immune system. Talk to it and encourage it to keep up the fight.

2. **Open yourself to humor, friendship, and love.**

Positive emotions strengthen the immune system. Fortunately, almost anything that helps you feel good about yourself helps you stay healthy.

Visualization

Visualization adds mental pictures to affirmations. Focus on your affirmation and start envisioning pictures that support it.

- Select one specific affirmation. For example, "My hands are flexible and pain-free."

- Develop a mental image of your affirmation. For example, for pain-free hands, imagine that a cool, soothing fluid is pouring over your hands, making them more and more flexible. Be as creative as you like, but keep it simple.

- Repeat the mental picture over and over. Combine several longer sessions with short replays of the visual picture throughout the day.

- Add positive self-talk and affirmations to the mental picture. If any doubts arise, dismiss them until after the exercise. This time is for positive thoughts only.

- Practice makes perfect. With daily visualizations, you will soon be creating mental pictures that help you meet your goals.

- Laugh. Life with a little humor mixed in is both richer and more healthy. Laughter increases creativity, reduces pain, and speeds healing. Keep an emergency laughter kit of funny videotapes, jokes, cartoons, and photographs. Put it with your first-aid supplies and keep it well-stocked.

- Seek out friends. Friendships are vital to good health. Close social ties help you recover more quickly from illness and lessen your risk of developing diseases ranging from arthritis to depression.

- Volunteer. People who volunteer live longer and enjoy life more than those who do not. By helping others, we satisfy a basic need within ourselves. Whether you volunteer for a local non-profit organization, or for the neighbor next door, when you lend someone a hand, you also receive a boost in your own mental wellness.

- Plant a plant and pet a pet. Plants and pets can be highly therapeutic. When people stroke and pet animals, blood pressure goes down and heart rate slows. Animals and plants also help us feel needed. As long as we are involved in caring for others, whether people, pets, or plants, we help our bodies remain healthy.

3. **Appeal to the Spirit.**

If you believe in a higher power, ask for support in your pursuit of healing and health. Faith, prayer, and spiritual beliefs can play an important role in recovery from illness.

Your sense of spiritual wellness can help you overcome personal trials and to accept conditions that cannot be changed. If it suits you to do so, use spiritual images in visualizations, affirmations, and expectations about your health and your life.

Growing Wiser: Mental Wellness in Later Life

Although some people complain about their age, few would trade age for youth. It would mean giving up wisdom.

Wisdom is one of life's greatest gifts. Cultures the world over recognize the wisdom of their elders. However, although growing wiser is part of the natural aging process, it is not inevitable.

Two Voices

There are two competing voices within each person. One voice takes the role of the "Naysayer," the doubter. This voice mutters, "You're too old. You're not useful. You're not wanted. You're getting dependent." The Naysayer tries to limit what we can do and what we can enjoy.

The second voice within us is the voice of the "Sage." This is the voice of experience that tells us, "You have

Growing Wiser - continued

lots to offer. You are needed. You can make it." The ability to hear and listen to the Sage within us is essential to mental wellness.

Unfortunately, for many people, the Sage becomes dominated by the Naysayer. Myths and negative expectations about aging work to muffle the Sage while they strengthen the voice of the Naysayer.

Refuse to be limited by negative stereotypes! The secret to developing your wisdom is simply to recognize the Sage within you. The Growing Wiser Formula will encourage the voice of your internal sage. Use the formula to help structure your thinking about any problem that may otherwise place limits on you.

Growing Wiser Formula

Step One: Understand the Facts

Wisdom needs information with which to work. Learn all you can about yourself and your problem.

Focus not just on the negative consequences, but also on the positive potential within you.

Step Two: Reject Unnecessary Limitations

Carefully probe any uncertainties identified in Step One. If you cannot prove a negative assumption that threatens to limit your life, reject it. You can, for example, accept the negative fact that you have arthritis while rejecting the idea that it will

restrict you unduly. Our legal system assumes that people are innocent until proven otherwise. Give yourself the same benefit of the doubt.

Step Three: Create Positive Expectations

The most important factor in overcoming a problem is whether you expect to overcome it. Positive expectations can be built around affirmations and visualizations of your health goal. When you have a clear vision of what you would like to happen, it is easier to take control of the problem.

Positive expectations also trigger the release of healing substances within your body. The brain releases hundreds of chemical messengers that affect the healing process. Once you replace unnecessary limitations with positive expectations, your problem is often half-solved.

Step Four: Develop an Action Plan

The other half of problem solving is being ready to act. An action plan will put you in control. It will help you get what you want and expect out of life.

An effective action plan includes these elements:

- It addresses a goal.

- It considers all available options.

- It is something you can visualize.

- It is easy to start.

- It recognizes barriers.

- It includes rewards.

- It encourages support.

- It can be accomplished one step at a time.

For more on mental wellness for older adults, see Resource S2 on page 351.

Winning Over Serious Illness

A feeling of hopelessness and despair often arrives hand-in-hand with a diagnosis of life-threatening illness. The best way to triumph over cancer, heart disease, diabetes, or any other serious illness is to shake that feeling of hopelessness and stay in control of your life.

- The Growing Wiser Formula on page 310 can help you stay in control. Carefully consider each of the four steps.

- Remember who you really are. Who you are does not change because of your diagnosis.

- Keep communication open with family and friends. Talking openly about your illness will help them, too.

- Gather your support network around you. Forget any notion about being a burden. Letting people help you helps them to feel good about themselves.

- Join a support group of other people coping with the same problem. Finding even one person who has overcome a problem similar to yours can raise your spirits and add to your confidence.

Lots of people win their struggles over serious illness, either by being cured or by not letting illness control their lives. While there are no guarantees, taking charge of your life will give both your body and your mind the best opportunity to be victorious.

A great oak is only a little nut
that held its ground.
Anonymous

23

Declaring Independence

You are the captain of your own ship, the chief executive of your own corporation, and the president of your own sovereign state.

As a human being, your most basic right is to independently control your own life. This chapter will help you to understand and protect that right.

At age 30, 40, or 50, there is no question about your right to make your own decisions. It is up to you to decide where you will live, what you will do, and what risks you will take. As long as you don't break the law, you are pretty much left alone to do as you please.

Unfortunately, the longer you live, the more others may want to influence decisions that affect your life. These others are usually your children, or other relatives that love and care for you. In their efforts to care for and protect your health, they can unintentionally compromise your right to independence.

So long as you are mentally competent, you have the right to retain control over the basic decisions of your life--where you live, how you will spend your money and what health services you will accept, for example. (By writing down your wishes on a statement called an advance directive, you can retain some control over health care decisions even if you are no longer competent. See page 316.)

Certainly, you may wish to listen to the suggestions of your loved ones; they can be great sources of information. Listen carefully to the suggestions and options offered you, think them over, and then, decide for yourself. Being assertive will help you stay in charge.

Assertiveness

Assertiveness is the art of speaking up for yourself and getting what you want, without infringing on the rights of others. As an assertive person, you

Assertiveness - continued

can exercise your rights without denying or violating the rights and feelings of others. You can learn to state your preferences in a way that others will take seriously.

Assertiveness is the middle ground between aggressiveness and passivity. If you choose aggressiveness, you may get what you want, but the price may be very high. If you get your way by offending others, you could lose friendship and respect.

Passivity, on the other hand, rarely gets you what you want. If you are overly passive, you will not make your needs or wishes known. As a result, others may make decisions for you that you would rather make yourself.

Passivity may cause you to lose confidence and respect for yourself. You may feel helpless, controlled, and bitter because you rarely get what you really want.

Assertiveness Basics

- Think carefully about what you want and what you need.

- Arrange for a time to discuss the subject.

- Write down what you want and then talk about your problem.

- Describe your feelings about the subject using "I" messages. Say "I feel upset" instead of "You upset me."

- Be very specific about what you want.

- Listen and respond to the other person's concerns. This will improve your chances for agreement.

Being assertive doesn't mean being hard, cruel, or impolite. It simply means being clear about what you want and saying what you mean. It often means negotiating and reaching a compromise. However, the compromise isn't one you're forced into-- you agree to it on the basis of what you want.

Your Assertiveness Rights

You have the right to express your feelings.

You have the right to be treated fairly.

You have the right to live your life as you see fit.

You have the right to decide not to assert yourself.

Independence at Home

At some point, many older people must decide whether or not to leave the family home. Your loved ones may suggest it. They may point out many factors which would make a new place look good: being closer to the children, better climate, less expense, easier to clean, etc.

When you consider these factors, you may decide you do want to move. If so, great! Start packing. On the other hand, you may enjoy your current home very much. You may have friends and neighbors whom you would miss if you moved. And, there is help available to deal with housecleaning, maintenance, and other tasks that may be becoming more difficult for you. If you prefer not to move, make it clear to everyone that you, and only you, will decide if and when you will move.

When they can no longer take care of their homes, some people believe their choices are limited. They agree to move in with their children or into a retirement community because they don't realize there are other options. While moving is the right choice for some people, it may not be the right choice for you. Take some time to explore all of the options.

Services for Independent Living

The best way to remain independent is to know when to ask for help. The following services are available in many communities to help people maximize their independence. You can find out more about services available in your community by calling your local senior center. Ask for their "Information and Referral" person.

Chore services: help with major housecleaning, yard work, and minor household repairs.

Congregate Housing/Retirement Homes: special apartment complexes that provide supportive environments for older adults. Residents have their own apartments. Some facilities provide meals in a central location and offer a variety of services, such as laundry, housekeeping, and personal care.

Congregate Meals: hot meals served at a central location, usually a senior center. Social activities are sometimes offered, too.

Friendly visitors: non-medical attendants who provide companionship and some supervision for a few hours. They do not usually provide any housekeeping or personal care services.

Home-delivered meals (also called "Meals-on-Wheels"): hot, nutritious meals delivered to the home, usually at lunch. Some groups also provide meals that can be warmed for dinner.

Home Health Aides: provide personal care (bathing, help in using the toilet) and basic health care. Home health aides can be very helpful during post-hospital recovery, or to help with caregiving. This service can be provided round-the-clock, or for a few hours a week.

Homemaker Services: non-medical care in the home, such as housekeeping, cooking, shopping, and laundry.

Independent Living - continued

Personal Emergency Response System (PERS): a transmitter, generally worn around the neck or on the wrist. When activated, the PERS automatically places a call for help to an emergency response center.

Skilled Home Care: professional nursing care provided in the home for more serious medical problems. Skilled home care can usually be provided as often as needed, and is often supplemented with personal care provided by aides. Physical, respiratory, speech, and occupational therapy services are also available in the home.

Senior Centers: sites where older people gather for meals, social activities, and educational programs.

Advance Directives: Extending Control Over Health Care Decisions

You can exercise control over health care decisions even if dementia or other problems erode your competence. An advance directive is a legal document that expresses your personal wishes for future decisions. Three types of advance directives are discussed here.

A Living Will is a simple document that states your wishes regarding life-sustaining measures or other medical treatment should you become unable to speak for yourself. Be very specific about the conditions under which you would or would not want

---

Long-term Care Insurance

Medicare and private health insurance do not cover nursing home services or extended periods of home health care. Long-term care insurance is designed to protect families from the high costs of custodial care. When shopping for a policy of this kind, look for:

- Allowance of benefits without requiring a prior hospital stay

- Premiums that do not increase because of age or health status

- Benefits for in-home care

- Guaranteed lifetime renewability

- Comprehensive coverage of all levels of long-term care

- Specific coverage for Parkinson's, Alzheimer's, and any other illness involving dementia

- A waiver of premiums while receiving benefits in a long-term care facility

- No waiting period for coverage of pre-exisiting conditions

---

certain kinds of treatment. Some states have a basic form to which you can add your own personal instructions.

A Living Will can be changed or revoked at any time. Be sure two witnesses sign the document and have it notarized. You do not need an attorney to write a Living Will, but legal advice may be helpful if your state's statutes are unclear or your state does not recognize Living Wills.

A Durable Power of Attorney for Health Care is a legal document that gives another person the authority to make health care decisions on your behalf if you are unable to do so. The person you choose should understand and respect your personal wishes about medical treatment. You may specify in the document how you would like such decisions to be made. A Durable Power of Attorney may also give another person the authority to make financial and other decisions, if you choose.

You must be mentally competent to execute a Durable Power of Attorney. For this reason, anyone who has a progressive brain disorder such as Parkinson's disease or Alzheimer's disease may wish to draw up this document as early as possible to avoid later difficulties when judgment becomes impaired.

A Conservatorship or **Guardianship** is used if a person has already become incapacitated. It may be the only way for someone else to assume control over that person's affairs. A conservator may make financial decisions and other personal decisions such as place of residence, consent for services, etc. A third

party may petition the court to ask that a conservator be appointed.

Each state has its own set of rules regarding advance directives. You may wish to consult with an attorney or your local hospital. Hospitals and long-term care facilities that receive Medicare or Medicaid are required to notify all patients of their rights to draw up advance directives stating their wishes about medical or surgical treatment.

Who's In Charge?

Sometimes, you may choose to let someone else take control of some parts of your life. The important thing is that **you** decide what areas of your life you will permit someone else to control. Do not allow other people to talk you into making decisions that you are not comfortable with, even if you think their intentions are good.

Independence has no age limit. You have the right to retain control of your life for as long as you live. There are many options available to help you keep your freedom and independence.

It is up to **you** to make decisions and seek out services that will help you stay independent as long as you wish. Just as you need to exercise your mind and body to keep them strong, you need to exercise your right to control your life.

You **can** control your own life. You **are** in charge.

One of the deep secrets of life
is that all that is really worth the doing
is what we do for others.
Lewis Carroll

24

Caregiver Secrets

There are three secrets to being a good caregiver:

- Take care of yourself first.

- Don't help too much.

- Don't do it alone.

This chapter will help you learn these secrets and how they can aid both you and the person for whom you care.

Caregiver Secret #1: Take Care of Yourself First

If you want to give good care, you have to take care of yourself first.

Caregivers tend to deny their own needs. This need-denial strategy may work fine for short-term caregiving. However, for long-term caregiving commitments, it inevitably leads to problems.

There are three things that happen when caregivers don't take good care of themselves:

1. They become ill.

2. They become depressed.

3. They "burn out" and stop providing care altogether.

These three things are bad for both the caregiver and the person receiving the care.

On the other hand, when caregivers take time to care for themselves, three good things happen:

1. They avoid health problems.

2. They feel better about themselves.

3. They have more energy and enthusiasm for helping others.

All You Have Is Time

Time is your most important resource. The problem is, you only have 24 hours of it in a day, and after you subtract the time you need to do your basic work and chores, there may be only a few hours left over. That is the time you have to spend

Caregiver Secret #1 - continued

exercising, preparing healthy meals, being with friends, and doing other things that you enjoy.

Caregiving requires a large commitment of time, perhaps all of the extra time you have for yourself. If that happens, problems can develop.

The best way to prevent the depression, frustration, and resentment that cause caregiver burnout is to hold back some time for yourself.

If you wait until all of your chores and caregiving tasks are done before doing things for yourself, you will wait a very long time. First, decide on the minimum amount of time necessary to meet your basic personal needs. Carve that time out of your schedule. Then, figure out how the chores and caregiving will get done.

---

10 Ways to Make Extra Time for Yourself

5 Ways that Don't Cost Money

- Trade a morning or an afternoon a week with another caregiver.

- Ask several relatives, friends, church members, or neighbors if each would relieve you for two to four hours per week on a regular schedule.

- Sign up for respite services. Some are available for no cost or for a voluntary donation.

- Barter for services...a loaf of bread for an hour of care.

- Use locking dutch doors to create a part of the house that is just for you--at least for a part of each day.

5 Ways that Can Cost Money

- Hire a teenager or older adult to stay with the person for a few hours each day.

- Sign up for homemaker or chore services. By saving a few hours of housekeeping, you might strengthen your more important caregiving skills.

- Sign up for a home-delivered meal service.

- Enroll the person in adult day care. Even a part-time placement for several hours per week can be helpful to both you and the person for whom you care.

- Hire a home health aide.

How to Take Care of Yourself

The biggest health threat to caregivers is depression. Maintaining a strong self-image is the most important thing that a caregiver can do to care for herself. Use self-care, extra support, and professional help as appropriate when the earliest signs of depression appear. See page 242 for suggestions.

Exercise can be a good energizer for both physical and emotional health. The guidelines in Chapter 19 can lead you on a path to fitness, one small step at a time.

Good nutrition is also important to caregiving. Tips in Chapter 20 can help you reduce fat and increase fiber and carbohydrates in your diet. You may discover that a good diet will give you more energy to carry you through each day. Don't feel you have to change too much at once. One small diet improvement at a time can make a big difference over a year's time.

Your need for stress management and relaxation increases during periods of caregiving. Chapter 21 can get you started on quick, easy-to-learn relaxation techniques that will help you deal with any frustrations and stresses that build up.

Take heart. You don't need to change everything at once. Just select any area of your health that you would like to improve. This book can help you move closer to your goal, one step at a time.

Caregiver Guilt

The people who provide the most care to others often feel the most guilt. There is an old saying, "Scratch guilt and you will find resentment."

When caregiving uses up all of your extra time, you may begin to feel frustrated and angry. This can lead to a cycle of help, frustration, and guilt that repeats itself over and over.

The best way to let go of guilt is to accept the fact that you just can't be everything to everyone all of the time.

- Acknowledge your limitations. If you try to do too much, frustration is inevitable.

- Prioritize your caregiving. Decide to do only what is most important. Refuse to feel guilty about unmade beds or dusty windows.

- Allow yourself to be less than perfect. Tell yourself that you are doing a good job at a very difficult task. Pat yourself on the back for your caregiving and reward yourself.

- Ask for help. Feeling guilty is often a sign that you need a break from your caregiving schedule. If your "guilt-o-meter" starts to increase, explore other options or ask friends and family to pitch in.

Caregiver Secret #2: Don't Help Too Much

The biggest mistake most caregivers make is providing too much care. Even if they don't admit it, people like to help themselves. Every time you provide care that could have been done by the one you are caring for, there is a double loss. First, your effort is wasted. Second, the person is denied an opportunity to help himself.

Help Them To Help Themselves

The caregiver's highest goal is to give the person the power and the permission to control as much of his life as possible. Every act your loved one makes toward maintaining independence is a victory for you as a caregiver.

Too often we get trapped in the role of a rescuer. We come to the person's rescue and expect to be rewarded with thanks and praise. Often, the thanks never come.

Too much rescuing teaches the one receiving care to be helpless. Eventually he will lose both the skills and the desire to do things for himself. Instead of rescuing, try to empower.

10 Ways to Empower the Person for Whom You Care

1. Expect more. People respond to expectations. If you expect someone to dress himself, care for his plants, or cook simple meals, he often will.

2. Limit your availability to help. If you are not always there to help, the person will be forced to do more for himself.

3. Simplify. For those with mild dementia, divide complex tasks into simpler parts: First, get out the cereal box; next get out the milk and the bowl, etc.

4. Make it easy. One of the most productive things a caregiver can do is to find tools that help the person to help himself. See Resource H1 on page 350.

5. Allow for mistakes. The hardest thing about letting someone do something for himself is knowing that you could do it better or faster. Mistakes are okay.

6. Reward both effort and results. Help the person feel good about doing things for himself.

7. Let him make as many decisions as he can, even about simple things like what to wear, what to eat, or when to go to bed. Your goal is to help him retain as much control over his life as possible.

8. Give him responsibility to care for something. Studies show that nursing home patients who are asked to care for pets or plants live longer and become more independent.

9. Match tasks with abilities. Actively identify the person's skills and try to match them with ways he can help himself.

10. Take acceptable risks. A few broken dishes or a few bruises are a small price to pay for letting someone explore what he can do for himself. You can't eliminate all risks without eliminating all opportunities.

Caring for a Person with Dementia

- If your loved one has been diagnosed as having Alzheimer's disease or another form of progressive dementia, discuss important matters like a will, a living will, and a durable power of attorney early when his judgment is best. See page 316.

- Be aware that confusion often increases around sundown. Don't plan any complicated activities for that time.

- Arrange for respite care. The primary caregiver's need for rest increases as dementia worsens. Regular breaks from caregiving will help give you the stamina you need to care for the person as long as possible. Family and friends can help but other options should be explored. See page 325.

- Recognize when placement in a caregiving facility becomes appropriate. When home care can no longer be provided safely or without harm to others, consider placement away from home.

Ask if the staff is particularly knowledgeable about dementia. Some facilities have special units designed for people who have dementing illnesses.

- See Resources D1-2 on page 349 for information on caring for a person with dementia. Also, contact the Alzheimer's Association at (800) 272-3900 for the chapter nearest you.

Caregiver Needs for Respite

If you can answer "yes" to one or more of the following questions, it's time to get more help.

- Do I feel overworked and exhausted?

- Do I feel dissatisfied with myself?

- Do I feel isolated?

- Do I feel depressed, resentful, angry, or worried?

- Do I feel that I have no time for myself?

- Do I have no time to exercise and rest?

- Do I have no time for fun with people outside of my family?

A Caregiver's Bill of Rights

I have the right to take care of myself. This is not an act of selfishness. It will give me the capability of taking better care of my relative.

I have the right to seek help from others even though my relative may object. I recognize the limits of my own endurance and strength.

I have the right to maintain facets of my own life that do not include the person I care for, just as I would if he or she were healthy. I know that I do everything that I reasonably can for this person, and I have the right to do some things just for myself.

I have the right to get angry, be depressed, and express other difficult feelings occasionally.

I have the right to reject any attempt by my relative (either conscious or unconscious) to manipulate me through guilt, anger, or depression.

I have the right to receive consideration, affection, forgiveness, and acceptance for what I do from my loved one for as long as I offer these qualities in return.

I have the right to take pride in what I am accomplishing and to applaud the courage it has sometimes taken to meet the needs of my relative.

I have the right to protect my individuality and my right to make a life for myself that will sustain me in the time when my relative no longer needs my full-time help.

I have the right to expect and demand that as new strides are made in finding resources to aid physically and mentally impaired older persons in our country, similar strides will be made toward aiding and supporting caregivers.

I have the right to:

_____

_____

_____

_____

_____

_____

_____

Caregiver Secret #3: Don't Do It Alone

Some caregivers live under the mistaken impression that they are the only available source of help. This is simply not true. In fact, if you want to be a good caregiver, start by knowing where to find help.

The following services help people remain as independent as possible. To learn whether these services are available in your community, look under "Senior Citizen Services" in your Yellow Pages. Your community or county office on aging should be listed. Also see pages 315-316 for more information.

- Chore services
- Congregate housing
- Congregate meals
- Friendly visitors
- Home-delivered meals
- Home health aides
- Homemaker services
- Senior centers
- Skilled home nursing care

Respite care may be the most important service for caregivers. Respite attendants provide short-term care for a few hours or a few days while you take a break.

Adult day care is usually offered during working hours, and is not always available on weekends It provides meals, personal care services, and social activities at a central location to people who need supervision.

Adult foster care or **board-and-care homes** are private homes in the community where older adults receive round-the-clock personal care, supervision, and meals. Some states require that board-and-care homes be licensed.

Nursing homes generally have two levels of care. Intermediate care includes assistance with toileting, dressing, and personal care for people without serious medical

Paying for Caregiving Services

Long-term nursing home and caregiver services are generally not covered by Medicare or private health insurance. However, if the need is related to a medical problem, short-term services are often eligible for reimbursement.

Many of the caregiver services listed here and in Chapter 23 are subsidized through federal and state funding. The coverage, subsidy, and eligibility vary from state to state. To learn what help is available to you, call your state office on aging. Many of these agencies have a toll-free number.

Caregiver Secret #3 - continued

conditions. Skilled nursing care is usually for people who have just come from the hospital, or others with medical conditions that require more intensive nursing care. Some facilities have special units for people with dementia.

Hospice programs provide social, personal, and medical services to terminally ill patients who wish to spend their remaining time at home or in a less formal medical facility.

Take Pride

Now that you know the three secrets of caregiving, you can see that they really aren't secrets at all. There is nothing magical or mysterious about being a good caregiver.

- Care for your own needs first--both your physical and mental health depend on it. Give yourself as much special attention as you give the person for whom you care.

- Help the person you care for to help himself--this is a gift both to you and to him.

- Recognize when you need extra help, and know where you can get it. A helping hand at the right time can make all the difference.

Take pride in being a caregiver. It is not easy, and those who do it are very special people. The three secrets of caregiving can help you feel good about yourself and the care you give.

A merry heart doeth good like a medicine.
Proverbs 17:22

25

Medication Management

What ever happened to "laughter is the best medicine?" While a positive attitude is more important to our health than perhaps we realize, it can't cure everything. Medicines now help to control many diseases that once were crippling or fatal. Arthritis, cancer, diabetes, high blood pressure, heart disease, and many other conditions now can be treated successfully with drugs. Used improperly, however, medications may cause problems and do more harm than good.

Good medication management begins in your doctor's office, when a prescription is written, but it doesn't stop there. This chapter includes tips on how to organize and take medications, as well as information on some common over-the-counter and prescription drugs. Guidelines for recognizing and avoiding problems caused by medications are also included.

Medications and Older Adults

Medications have special importance for older adults. As a group, people over age 50 receive more prescriptions than people of other ages. Many older people are taking unnecessary or even harmful medications. Not only is this bad for one's health, it is also painful to the wallet!

Drugs are expensive and the costs of several prescriptions add up quickly. Successful medication management will not only prevent adverse health effects, but will save money as well.

Be Smart About Pills

Studies have shown that two-thirds of the prescriptions written for older people are unnecessary, too risky, or the wrong dose. Keep the following items in mind to make sure you are not taking unneeded drugs.

- Discuss all medication decisions with your doctor.

Medications - continued

- Consider other options for treating an illness besides medication. Exercise, diet changes, and stress management can provide many of the benefits of drugs.

- Start low, go slow. Ask your doctor if you can begin new medications at a low dose and increase only as needed. Many drugs are tested on young adults. Older adults often need a lower dose.

You and Your Medications

Ask Your Doctor:

- What is the name of this drug? What are the brand names?

- Why is it being prescribed? What will it do for me?

- What are the side effects? Will it interact with my other medications? (Take a list of all your drugs.)

- Will a lower dose provide the same benefit?

- Are there any risks if I try a non-drug treatment first?

- Is a generic equivalent available?

- Do you have samples I can take for a trial period?

- What are the directions for use?

- When can I stop taking the drug?

Ask Your Pharmacist:

- How often do I take it? Are there instructions for use?

- What side effects may occur? How do I recognize them?

- Are there special precautions, such as avoiding certain foods, alcohol, other medications, or the sun?

- Are there storage instructions?

- What if I miss a dose?

- Can you help me with:

  - Color-coded containers to help with organization

  - Easy-open caps and large print labels

  - Maintaining a record of my medications

  - Delivery to my home

  - 24-hour emergency service

- Re-evaluate your medications regularly. Ask your doctor if there are any you can safely stop taking.

- Don't make any change in the number or kind of medications you take without consulting your doctor first.

- Put a pharmacist on your health care team. Pharmacists are good people to go to with questions about prescription and over-the-counter medications.

Organize Your Pills

Good medication management also means organizing your bottles and pills. Avoid confusion and mistakes by following these simple steps:

- Take your medication record to each doctor visit.

- Keep accurate, up-to-date records on all medications. Use a form like the one on page 342. Include any over-the-counter medications, such as aspirin or laxatives.

- Store medications properly.

  ○ Keep medications in a cool, dry place. Hot, steamy bathrooms cause medications to lose their strength. Some drugs need refrigeration. Ask your pharmacist.

  ○ Keep drugs in their original containers. Clearly label any drugs that you put in different bottles.

  ○ Inspect your medications at least once a year. Dispose of expired, unused, unlabeled, and discolored drugs by flushing them down the toilet.

Simplify Your Pill Schedule

Taking three or four different drugs each day according to different schedules can be very confusing. Develop a system to keep track of when and how you take each medication.

- Show your primary doctor a complete list of the drugs you take and the times you now take them. Ask if he or she could help you simplify the schedule so that you take your pills only once or twice a day.

- List your medication schedule on a daily planner that has spaces for hourly notations. Post it in a prominent place near your medicine cabinet. Take it with you when you travel.

- Use a pillbox designed to hold a week's worth of pills. You can also label empty egg cartons and use them to organize a day's or week's worth of medications.

- Post reminders near clocks or on the bathroom mirror to help keep you on schedule.

- Take medications with a full glass of water, unless instructed otherwise. Avoid lying down soon after

Pill Schedule - continued

taking your pills, as they may get stuck in your esophagus and cause pain.

- Don't crush or mix medications into hot liquids or foods. The drug may lose its effectiveness.

- Never take any prescription or over-the-counter medication with alcohol.

Spend Less Money on Pills

Prescription medications are very expensive. Besides avoiding unneeded drugs, you can cut your medication costs in these ways:

- Buy generic drugs. They are chemically equivalent to name-brand drugs, but are usually cheaper. Ask your doctor if generic forms of your medications are available and appropriate for you.

- Compare prices between several pharmacies. It may be worth paying a little more if you are comfortable with the pharmacist, but do shop around. Prices can vary widely.

- Ask your doctor for samples of newly prescribed medications, or ask your pharmacist to fill only the first week's worth of pills. If the medication has to be changed

Mail-Order or the Local Pharmacy?

If you regularly take the same medications, buying them through a mail-order pharmacy may save money. However, before you place your order, talk with your local pharmacist. Most pharmacies offer a senior citizen discount and many compete well with mail-order prices. Your local pharmacy also offers a number of valuable services:

- Convenience and immediate availability

- The pharmacist's professional advice

- Personal service

- The ability to monitor all of your prescriptions for possible interactions

Before you switch to a mail-order drug company, be sure that the savings are worth the other services that you may be giving up.

later, you won't have wasted the price of the full prescription.

- Consider buying regularly used, high-cost drugs from mail-order pharmacies.

Over-the-Counter (OTC) Medications

An over-the-counter (OTC) medication is any drug that can be purchased without a physician's prescription. However, don't assume that all OTC drugs are safe for you. These drugs can interact with other medications and can sometimes create serious health problems.

Carefully read the label of any over-the-counter drug you are using, and ask your pharmacist for help in finding the one best suited to your needs.

Some of the most common OTCs include:

- Antacids

- Anti-diarrheals

- Cold remedies

- Laxatives

- Pain relievers, such as aspirin, acetaminophen, and ibuprofen

These drugs can be very helpful when used properly, but can also create serious problems if used incorrectly. The following tips will help you use these common OTC drugs wisely and safely. In some cases, you may find that you don't need to take them at all.

Antacids

Antacids are taken to reduce indigestion or heartburn caused by excess stomach acid. While they are safe if used occasionally, antacids may cause problems if taken regularly.

There are several kinds of antacids. Get to know what ingredients are in each type so that you can avoid any adverse effects.

- Sodium bicarbonate antacids (Alka-Seltzer and Bromo Seltzer) contain baking soda. If you have high blood pressure, or if you are on a salt-restricted diet, avoid these antacids because of their high sodium content. If used too frequently, they may interfere with kidney or heart function.

- Calcium carbonate antacids (TUMS, Alka-2) are sometimes used as calcium supplements. A single tablet provides 20% of the recommended dietary allowance of calcium. However, these products may cause constipation. Limit use to only four or five tablets per day if you are taking them as a calcium supplement.

- Aluminum-based antacids (Amphojel) are less potent and work more slowly than other products. Some may cause calcium depletion and should not be taken by postmenopausal women. Check with your doctor before using aluminum antacids if you have kidney problems.

- Magnesium compounds (Phillip's Milk of Magnesia) may cause diarrhea.

OTC Medications - continued

- Aluminum-magnesium antacids (Maalox, Di-Gel, Mylanta, Riopan) are generally less likely to cause constipation or diarrhea than aluminum-only or magnesium-only antacids.

Antacid Precautions

- Try to eliminate the cause of frequent heartburn instead of taking antacids regularly. Stop smoking and cut down on alcohol, caffeine, and fatty foods. See Heartburn on page 107.

- Consult your doctor or pharmacist before taking an antacid if you take other medications. Antacids may interfere with the absorption and action of some drugs, such as antibiotics, digitalis, and anti-coagulants. Also consult your doctor if you have ulcers or kidney problems.

- Call a health professional immediately if your heartburn is severe and accompanied by chest pain, shortness of breath, nausea, vomiting, fainting, or sweating. This may signal a heart attack.

Anti-diarrheal Preparations

Because diarrhea often helps to rid your body of an infection, try to avoid using anti-diarrheal medications for the first six hours. Then, use only if the diarrhea is causing cramping and pain.

There are two types of anti-diarrheal drugs: those that thicken the stool and those that slow intestinal spasms.

The thickening mixtures contain clay or fruit pectin and absorb the bacteria and toxins in the intestine. Although they are safe in that they do not go into the system, these anti-diarrheals also absorb bacteria needed in digestion. Their continued use is not advised.

Be sure to take a large enough dose. Anti-diarrheal preparations should be taken until the stool thickens, then stopped immediately to avoid constipation.

Antispasmodic anti-diarrheal products stop the spasm of the intestine. Loperamide (Imodium A-D) is an example of this type of preparation. Donnagel and Parepectolin contain both thickening and anti-spasmodic ingredients.

Anti-diarrheal Precautions

- Do not take any anti-diarrheal product if you have glaucoma, kidney or liver disease, or prostate problems.

- Replace depleted body fluids. Diarrhea causes your body to lose fluids and salts (called electrolytes), which may cause dehydration. When you have diarrhea, avoid drinking or eating anything for a few hours, but after that, drink plenty of extra liquids. You can buy Gatorade at the supermarket or Lytren at the pharmacy;

both are good solutions to replace needed fluids or salts. You can also make an inexpensive home-made electrolyte solution. Mix:

- 1 quart water

- 1/2 teaspoon baking soda

- 1/2 teaspoon table salt

- 2 tablespoons sugar

- If available, add 1/4 teaspoon salt substitute ("Lite Salt")

Cold Medications

In general, if you take drugs for your cold, you'll get better in about a week. If you take nothing, you'll get better in about seven days. Rest and liquids are probably the best treatment for a cold. Antibiotics will not help. However, medications are helpful in relieving some cold symptoms.

Antihistamines

Antihistamines are commonly used to treat allergy symptoms, and they are also found in most cold medications. They are frequently combined with a decongestant. Antihistamines dry up mucous membranes, and may make the person with a runny nose more comfortable, whether the cause is a cold or an allergy.

It is usually best to take only single-ingredient cold preparations. For example, if your most troublesome symptom is a runny nose, you should not take a drug that contains a decongestant, too.

Dristan, Coricidin, and Triaminic are cold preparations that contain both decongestants and antihistamines.

Chlor-Trimeton (chlorpheniramine) and Benadryl (diphenhydramine) are single-ingredient antihistamine products.

Antihistamine Precautions

The value of antihistamines in treating cold symptoms is under debate. Antihistamines dry all mucous membranes. Drying the mucous membranes may prolong a cold, since moist membranes help to filter the air.

- Drink extra fluids when taking cold medications.

- Don't drive or operate machinery. Antihistamines may cause dizziness, drowsiness, and abnormally low blood pressure in older adults. They may also cause increased activity in some people. Don't take antihistamines:

  - If you have asthma, glaucoma, an enlarged prostate gland, ulcers, or hypertension.

  - If you are taking anti-depressant medications, sedatives, hypnotics, or tranquilizers.

- Antihistamines can interact with other medications. Ask your pharmacist to help you choose a cold medicine that will not react with your other drugs.

Decongestants

Decongestants make breathing easier by shrinking swollen mucous membranes in the nose and allowing air to pass through the nose. They also help relieve runny nose and postnasal drip, which can cause a sore throat.

Decongestants can be taken orally or used as nose drops or sprays. Oral decongestants (pills) are probably more effective and provide longer relief. Pseudoephedrine (Sudafed) is an OTC oral decongestant.

Sprays and drops provide immediate but temporary relief. Phenylephrine (Neo-synephrine) is an effective nasal spray for temporary relief. Sprays and drops have the added benefit that they are less likely than oral decongestants to interact with other drugs.

Decongestant Precautions

- If you have asthma, high blood pressure, heart disease, diabetes, urinary retention, glaucoma, or thyroid disease, you should use decongestants only as directed by a physician.

- Decongestants can cause drowsiness or increased activity in some people. Some brands also interfere with sleep.

- Too much decongestant can cause hallucinations and convulsions, and may depress central nervous system functions in older people.

Saline Nose Drops

The safest nasal drop for a stuffy nose is home-made saline solution. Saline nose drops will not cause a rebound effect. They keep nasal tissues moist so they can filter the air.

Mix 1/4 teaspoon salt in 1 cup distilled water (too much salt will dry nasal membranes).

Place the solution in a clean bottle with a dropper (available at drugstores). Use as necessary. Discard and make a fresh solution weekly.

To insert drops, lie down with your head hanging over the side of the bed. This helps the drops get farther back. Try to prevent the dropper from touching your nose.

Use long-acting formulas only as directed.

- Do not use medicated nasal sprays or drops for more than three days nor more than three times a day. Continued use can lead to a "rebound effect": the mucous membranes swell as with a cold.

Cough Preparations

Coughing is your body's way of getting foreign substances, phlegm, and mucus out of your respiratory tract. Coughs are often useful and you usually don't want to eliminate them. Sometimes, though, coughs are severe enough to impair breathing or prevent rest.

There are two kinds of cough preparations. **Expectorants** help thin the mucus, making it easier to "bring up." Robitussin is an expectorant cough syrup. Look for products containing guaifenesin.

Suppressants are used to control or suppress a nagging cough. They subdue the cough reflex and work best for the dry, hacking cough that keeps you awake.

Look for suppressant medications containing dextromethorphan, such as Robitussin-DM.

Water and other liquids, such as fruit juices, are probably the best cough syrups. They help soothe the throat, and also moisten and thin mucus so that it can be coughed up more easily.

You can make a simple and soothing cough syrup at home by mixing one part lemon juice with two parts honey. Use as often as needed.

Cough drops may soothe the throat, but so will water or juice, which also add needed fluids. Medicated drops are generally no more effective than ordinary candy drops.

Cough Suppressant Precautions

- Use with caution if you have chronic respiratory problems; cough suppressants can stifle breathing. Use care when giving cough suppressants to the very old or frail.

- Do not take cough medications containing dextromethorphan if you are taking anti-depressant medications.

- Do not use cough suppressants if you have constipation problems.

- Read the label so you know what ingredients you are taking. Some cough preparations contain a large percentage of alcohol; others contain codeine. There are many choices. Ask your pharmacist to advise you.

- Call a health professional if any cough persists for more than 7 to 10 days without improvement.

Laxatives

A laxative is a compound that eases the passage and elimination of bowel movements. They are overused by many people. You can become dependent on laxatives if you use them incorrectly.

Water is the simplest and best laxative. Simply drinking more water is the first treatment to try for constipation. Also, try increasing your fiber intake (whole grains, raw vegetables, beans, and fruits such as prunes and apples). More dietary fiber and increased physical activity may provide relief.

Laxative Precautions

- Take any laxative with plenty of water or other liquids.

Laxatives - continued

- Do not use mineral oil as a laxative for more than a few days. It interferes with the body's absorption of vitamins. Also, it can leak from the anus and be inconvenient.

- Do not take laxatives regularly. Over-use of laxatives decreases tone and sensation in the large intestine, causing dependence on the laxative.

- Regular use of some laxatives (Correctol, Ex-Lax, Feen-A-Mint) may interfere with your body's absorption of vitamin D and calcium, which may weaken your bones. See page 99 for more home treatment tips for constipation.

Pain Relievers: Aspirin, Acetaminophen and Ibuprofen

Aspirin is widely used for relieving pain and reducing fever in adults. It also relieves minor itching, reduces swelling and inflammation, and is valuable for treating arthritis.

Aspirin Precautions

Although it seems familiar and safe, aspirin is a very powerful drug. Older adults need to be especially cautious of the potential dangers and side effects of aspirin:

- Aspirin can irritate the stomach lining, causing bleeding or ulcers. If you find that aspirin upsets your stomach, try a coated brand, such as Ecotrin. However, coated aspirin may not relieve pain as effectively as uncoated. Talk with your doctor or pharmacist to determine what will work best for you.

- Some people are allergic to aspirin. (These people may also be allergic to ibuprofen.)

- Do not take aspirin:

  ○ If suffering from gout

  ○ If taking blood thinners (anticoagulants)

  ○ For a hangover

- High doses may result in aspirin poisoning (salicylism). Symptoms of aspirin poisoning include:

  ○ Ringing in the ears

  ○ Visual disturbances

  ○ Nausea

  ○ Dizziness

  ○ Rapid, deep breathing

Stop taking aspirin and call a health professional if any of these symptoms occur.

Acetaminophen (Tylenol, etc.) is less likely than aspirin to cause an allergic reaction or stomach irritation. However, acetaminophen does not have the anti-inflammatory properties of aspirin and is not recommended for treatment of arthritis pain. It is useful as a mild pain reliever for cold and flu symptoms or headaches.

Ibuprofen (Advil, Nuprin, etc.) is another pain reliever that is available over-the-counter. Ibuprofen does not cause ringing in the ears like aspirin, but it may cause stomach irritation, nausea, and heartburn. It should also be used with caution by people taking blood-thinners (anti-coagulants). Ibuprofen, like aspirin, is an anti-inflammatory. Prescription-strength ibuprofen is available through your doctor.

Prescription Medications

There are thousands of different prescription drugs, used to treat hundreds of different medical conditions. Your best sources of information about your prescription medications are your doctor and your pharmacist. Look to them to answer your questions about medications. There are also good books available that contain information on many different prescription drugs. See Resources Q1-2 on page 351.

Guidelines for taking every kind of prescription medication could fill several books. Two common types are covered here: antibiotics and minor tranquilizers/sleeping pills.

Antibiotics

Antibiotics are prescription drugs that kill bacteria. They are only effective against bacteria, and have no effect on viruses. Antibiotics will not cure the common cold, influenza, or any other viral illness.

Antibiotics kill all the bacteria in the body that are sensitive to them--including those that help your body. Thus, the bacterial balance in your body may be destroyed while you are taking an antibiotic, and you may develop stomach upset, a vaginal infection, or some other problem.

You should take antibiotics only when needed to fight a bacterial infection. There are several reasons for this. First, antibiotics can cause many side effects. Most of these are mild, but they can be severe. If you have any unexpected reaction to an antibiotic, tell your health professional before another antibiotic is prescribed.

Second, bacteria build resistance to antibiotics. An antibiotic may become less effective if it is used too often.

Third, some people are allergic to antibiotics and may experience severe, life-threatening reactions.

Fourth, if the antibiotic is not useful in fighting the infection, why waste your time, money, energy, and health?

When you and your health professional have decided that an antibiotic is necessary, follow the instructions with the prescription carefully.

- Take the whole dose for as many days as prescribed, unless you

Antibiotic					

Antibiotic	Not affected by food	Empty stomach: 1 hr before or 2 hrs after meals	With meals	Not with milk	Not with antacids
Ampicillin		✓			
Amoxicillin	✓				
Augmentin	✓				
Cephalosporins:					
Cefaclor (Ceclor)	✓				
Cefadroxil (Duricef)	✓				
Cephalexin (Keflex)	✓				
Cephradine (Velocef)	✓				
CIPRO	✓				
Dicloxacillin (Dynapen)		✓			
Doxycycline			✓		✓
Erythromycin:					
E-Mycin, Ery-Tab	✓				
ERYC		✓			
Ilosone			✓		
Minocycline (Minocin)					✓
Nitrofurantoin			✓		
Penicillin G		✓			
Penicillin VK	✓				
Tetracycline		✓		✓	✓
Bactrim, Septra	✓				

Antibiotics - continued

have severe unexpected side effects. Antibiotics kill off many bacteria quite quickly, so you may feel better in a few days. If you stop too soon, it is possible that only the weaker bacteria will have been eliminated, and the stronger ones will survive and flourish.

- Be sure you understand any special instructions about taking the medication. These should be printed on the label, but double check with your physician and pharmacist. The chart on page 338 lists many antibiotics and advice for their use.

- Store antibiotics in a dry, cool place. They will usually keep their potency for about a year. However, most are prescribed only for a specific illness in an amount needed to cure that illness. Liquid antibiotics are always dated. Most are good for two weeks if refrigerated, or one week if kept at room temperature.

- Never give an antibiotic prescribed for one person to another.

- Do not take an antibiotic for another illness without a health professional's instructions.

Minor Tranquilizers and Sleeping Pills

Minor tranquilizers like Valium, Librium, Xanax, and Tranxene, and sleeping pills like Dalmane, Restoril, and Halcion are widely prescribed for older adults. However, these drugs can cause problems, for example, memory loss, mental impairment, addiction, and injuries from falls due to drug-induced unsteadiness.

Minor tranquilizers can be effective when prescribed for short periods of time. However, continued use is of questionable value and introduces the risk of addiction and mental impairment.

Sleeping pills rarely provide long-term relief. They may help for a few days or even a few weeks, but using sleeping pills for more than a month generally causes more sleep problems than the pills solve. For other approaches to sleep problems, see page 251.

If you have been taking minor tranquilizers or sleeping pills for a while, talk with your doctor about discontinuing the drugs or reducing their dosage. Be sure to report any experiences you have had with unsteadiness, dizziness, or memory problems. These adverse effects of drugs are too often thought to be normal signs of aging.

Medication Problems

As the body ages, it becomes more susceptible to medication-related problems. One in five older adults

Medication Problems - cont'd

has experienced an adverse drug reaction to a prescription medication.

Aging brings on changes in the stomach, circulatory system, kidneys, and body composition. These changes affect the body's absorption, use, and excretion of medications. Drugs stay in the system longer, sometimes reaching very high concentrations.

Several different kinds of adverse medication reactions can occur:

Drug-drug interactions--two or more prescription or over-the-counter drugs mixing in the body and causing an adverse reaction. The symptoms can be severe and may be misdiagnosed as a new illness.

Drug-food interactions--medications reacting with food. Some drugs work best when taken with food, but others should be taken on an empty stomach. Some drug-food reactions can cause serious symptoms.

Over-medication--sometimes the full adult dose of a medication is too high for people over age 60. Too much of a drug is very dangerous.

Addiction--use of some medications over time leads to dependence on them and severe reactions if they are withdrawn suddenly. Narcotics, tranquilizers, and barbiturates should all be used with care to avoid addiction. See page 244.

Side effects--predictable, but unpleasant reactions to a drug. They are not usually serious, but can be inconvenient. In some people, they are severe and dangerous.

Adverse Drug Reactions

Side effects, drug-drug and food-drug interactions, over-medication, and addiction may cause:

- Nausea, indigestion, vomiting

- Constipation, diarrhea, incontinence, or difficulty urinating

- Edema (swelling)

- Dry mouth

- Headache, dizziness, ringing in the ears, or blurred vision

- Confusion, forgetfulness, disorientation, drowsiness, or depression

- Difficulty sleeping, irritability, or nervousness

- Difficulty breathing

- Rashes, bruising, and bleeding problems

Don't assume any symptom is a normal side effect or "just part of getting older." Call your doctor or pharmacist anytime you think your medicines are making you sick.

Prevention

- Develop a system for keeping track of your pill schedule. See page 329.

- Review your medications with your doctor often. See "You and Your Medications" on page 328.

- Review OTC drugs with your pharmacist. See "You and Your Medications" on page 328.

- Show a list of all the medications you take at every doctor visit.

- Tell your doctor and pharmacist about any allergies you have to medications.

- Never take a prescription that was written for another person. Don't share your medications with anyone. A drug that works wonders for you might be harmful to someone else.

Home Treatment

Sometimes, despite your best efforts, you will have an adverse reaction to a medication. Do not ignore symptoms that you suspect a drug has caused. They may be dangerous; even mild symptoms can cause serious problems.

- Keep a record of any symptom or side effect you have, even if it is minor. Show it to your doctor.

When to Call a Health Professional

- If any symptom, such as vomiting, breathing difficulties, headache, confusion, or drowsiness is severe or persistent.

- If symptoms develop soon after you have started taking a new medication, or after eating a certain food.

- If symptoms such as forgetfulness, depression, confusion, or fatigue develop slowly over a period of weeks or months. Some adverse drug effects take a while to show up.

- If you suspect that a symptom is related to an alcohol-drug interaction.

- When a mild symptom, such as dry mouth or constipation, interferes with your enjoyment of life.

Keep Track of all Medications

All medications, both prescription and over-the-counter, can have a powerful impact on your physical and mental health. Keep a medical record at home of all the drugs you use. See page 342 for a handy form.

Medication Record

Name: _____

Medication and Dose	Doctor/Date Prescribed	Color, Size, Shape	Purpose	Times Taken	Notes
(Example) Ampicillin 350 mg	Jacoby 4-15-92	blue and grey capsule	sinus infection	every 6 hours	Take on empty stomach.

Be prepared.
Boy Scout Motto

26

Your Home Health Center

Who provides most of the care for your health problems? Chances are, it's you. If you have the right tools, medicines, supplies, and information, you can do a better job. This chapter will help you to prepare your own home health center. The next time a health problem comes up, you will be ready!

Use the information on tools, supplies, medications, and books in this chapter to keep your home health center well-stocked. Store all your self-care resources in a central location. A large drawer in the bedroom or family room is a good place. You might also use a plastic tackle or sewing box to keep your supplies portable.

Self-Care Tools

Self-care tools are the basic equipment of your home health center.

Self-Care Tools

Keep these on hand:

- Blood pressure cuff
- Cold pack
- Dental mirror
- Eyedropper
- Heating pad
- Humidifier/Vaporizer
- Medicine spoon
- Nail clippers
- Scissors
- Stethoscope
- Thermometer
- Tweezers

Self-Care Tools - continued

Cold Pack

A cold pack is a plastic envelope filled with gel that remains flexible at very cold temperatures. Buy two cold packs at your pharmacy and keep them in the freezer. Use them for bumps, bruises, back sprains, turned ankles, sore joints, or any other health problem that calls for ice. A cold pack is more convenient than ice. It may become the self-care tool you use the most.

Humidifiers and Vaporizers

Humidifiers and vaporizers add moisture to the air. A humidifier produces a cool mist and a vaporizer puts out hot steam.

A humidifier has several advantages: it can't burn you; it makes tinier particles of water that get into your respiratory system better; it can't hurt the furniture; and, the cool mist is more comfortable than hot steam.

However, humidifiers are noisy, and they need to be cleaned and disinfected after each use. This is especially important for people who have mold allergies.

A vaporizer's hot steam may feel good when you have a cold, but the hot water can burn anyone who overturns it or gets too close. Whichever you choose, a humidifier or vaporizer will be an important self-care tool. They increase the humidity in the air, making it less drying to your mouth, throat, and nose.

Humidity in the air can help to soothe a scratchy throat, ease a dry, hacking cough, and make it easier for someone with a stuffy nose to breathe. Added humidity will make your home more comfortable, especially in the winter when dry air is a problem.

Medicine Spoon

A medicine spoon makes it easier to give the right dose of liquid medicine. It is a transparent tube with markings for typical liquid dosage amounts. Medicine spoons are convenient if you frequently take liquid prescription or over-the-counter medications. Buy one at your pharmacy.

Stethoscope and Blood Pressure Cuff (Sphygmomanometer)

If you have hypertension, it's a good idea to have both a stethoscope and a blood pressure cuff to monitor your blood pressure regularly.

For a stethoscope, purchase the flat diaphragm model rather than the bell-shaped one. The flat surface makes it easier for you to hear.

Blood pressure cuffs come in many models. If you have difficulty reading the gauge on a regular cuff, look for one attached to an upright mercury column, or an electronic digital model. Ask your pharmacist to recommend a blood pressure kit and show you how to use it.

Thermometer

Buy a thermometer with easy-to-read markings. Digital electronic thermometers are accurate and easy to read. Temperature strips are very convenient and safe, but are not as accurate as mercury or electronic thermometers.

Rectal thermometers with enlarged bulbs are helpful if the person cannot hold an oral thermometer in his mouth. Do not use a rectal thermometer if the person is confused or uncooperative.

Assistive Devices

If your hands and other body parts aren't as nimble as they used to be, consider assistive devices. They can help you with meal preparation, personal care, housekeeping, hobbies, and other activities. See Resource H1 on page 350 for a catalog of assistive devices.

OTC Products for Home Use

Keep some over-the-counter (OTC) products at home in case they are needed. Buy others only after symptoms develop. The chart on page 346 lists common health problems and suggestions for OTC products to treat them. For more information about OTC drugs, see page 331.

Home Medical Tests

Many common medical laboratory tests are now available in home kits. When combined with regular visits to your health professional, these home tests can help you to monitor your health, and in some cases, detect problems early.

Self-Care Supplies

Keep these on hand:

- Dental disclosing tablets

- Dental floss

- Adhesive strips ("Band-aids") in assorted sizes

- Adhesive tape -- one inch wide

- Butterfly bandages

- Sterile gauze pads -- two inches square

- Elastic ("Ace") bandage -- three inches wide

- Roll of gauze bandage -- two inches wide

- Cotton balls

- Safety pins

Home medical tests must be very accurate (over 95 percent) to be approved by the Food and Drug Administration. However, they must be used correctly to give such accurate results. Follow the package directions exactly. If you have questions, ask your pharmacist, or check the label for the company's toll-free phone number to call.

Home medical tests are especially helpful if you have a chronic condition that requires frequent monitoring, such as diabetes, asthma, or

OTC Products for Home Use

Problem	OTC Product (example)	Comments
Allergy	Antihistamines Chlor-Trimeton	To help dry mucous membranes. Also helpful for itching. See page 333.
Colds	Antihistamines; decongestants	See page 333 for precautions.
Constipation	Laxatives (Metamucil)	Avoid long-term or regular use. See page 335.
Cough, non-productive	Suppressants (Robitussin-DM)	To suppress the cough reflex. See page 335.
Cough, productive	Expectorants (Robitussin)	To thin and help clear the mucus. See page 335 for precautions.
Diarrhea	Anti-diarrheal (Kaopectate)	Avoid long-term use. See page 332.
Dry skin	Petroleum jelly (Vaseline)	Few side effects, inexpensive. See page 186.
Indigestion	Antacid (TUMS, Maalox)	Avoid long-term use. See page 331.
Itching	Hydrocortisone cream (Cortaid)	Antihistamines are also helpful. See page 186.
Pain, fever, inflammation	Aspirin or ibuprofen	Help to reduce swelling. May cause stomach upset. Not for children. See page 336.
	Acetaminophen	Pain relief; no anti-inflammatory effect; less stomach irritation. Safe for children. See page 336.
Scrapes, skin infections	Antibiotic creams (Bacitracin)	Keep creams cool and dry. Discard if out-of-date.

Home Medical Tests - continued

hypertension. Ask your doctor which home medical tests would be appropriate for your use. Some common tests are described below.

A more detailed description of these tests is included in the **Complete Guide to Medical Tests**. See Resource A1 on page 348.

Home Urinalysis

Some of the more common medical lab tests done on urine can also be done at home. Home urinalysis can help you monitor the progression of an illness or the effectiveness of a treatment. It is also useful if you have liver or kidney disease, diabetes, or if you have frequent urinary tract infections.

Home Blood Glucose Monitoring

If you have diabetes, you may already be monitoring your blood sugar levels using a finger prick and a test strip and/or an electronic monitor.

This test should always be used under a doctor's supervision, and you should never adjust your insulin dose based on a single abnormal test, unless your doctor has specifically instructed you to do so. Check with your doctor if you have symptoms of abnormal blood sugar levels, even if the test is normal. See page 125.

Home Blood Pressure Monitoring

If you have hypertension, it may be both expensive and inconvenient for you to visit your doctor for regular blood pressure checks. However, it is important that you monitor your blood pressure frequently. Blood pressure testing can be done easily at home with a little instruction.

By checking your blood pressure at home, when you are relaxed, you will be able to track changes due to your home treatment and medications.

- Do not make any changes to your medications based on your home blood pressure readings without consulting your doctor.

- Always check your blood pressure at the same time of day. Usually, blood pressure is lowest in the morning and rises during the day.

- For the most accurate reading, take the average of three readings, taken five to ten minutes apart.

Home Test for Blood in Stool

The fecal occult blood test can detect hidden blood in the stool, which may indicate colon cancer. If you have a family history of colon cancer, ask your doctor about screening. If your pharmacy does not stock the test, ask the pharmacist to order it for you.

This test is very sensitive to blood from other sources, such as bleeding gums, ulcers, and red meat in your diet. Be sure to follow the package instructions exactly, and report all positive results to your doctor.

Home Medical Records

Your home health center is a good place to keep your family's medical records, too. A three-ring binder or wire-bound notebook with dividers for each member of the family is helpful.

Each person should have a cover sheet listing:

- Diagnosed chronic conditions--arthritis, asthma, diabetes, high blood pressure

- Any known drug allergies

- Information that would be vital in an emergency--does the person have a pacemaker, a hearing aid, diabetes, epilepsy, or is he or she deaf or blind?

- Name and phone number of primary physician

Other important information that should be put on additional pages:

- An up-to-date list of medications. Include all the information shown in the sample chart on page 342.

- Immunization records--influenza, pneumococcal, tetanus

- Health screening results--blood pressure, cholesterol, vision, hearing

- Records of major illnesses and injuries, such as pneumonia, bronchitis, broken bones, or major infections

- Records of any major surgical procedures and hospitalizations

Your Home Health Library: Self-Care Resources

The most important self-care resource for the home is good information. Many of the resources listed below are available at your local bookstore or public library. If not, ask the bookstore to order the ones you want.

A. Three Books Every Home Should Have

1. H.W. Griffith, MD. *Complete Guide to Medical Tests*, Tucson, AZ: Fisher Books, 1988.

2. M. Mettler and D.W. Kemper. *Healthwise for Life*, Healthwise, 1992. Available from Healthwise, Inc., P.O. Box 1989, Boise, ID 83701, (208) 345-1161.

3. J. W. Long, M.D. *The Essential Guide to Prescription Drugs, 1992: Everything You Need to Know for Safe Drug Use*, New York, NY: Harper Collins Publishers, 1992.

B. General Purpose Resources

1. The Dartmouth Institute for Better Health. *Medical and Health Guide for People Over Fifty*, Glenview, IL: Scott, Foresman, and Company, 1986. Available from the American Association of Retired Persons, 601 E Street, NW, Washington, DC 20049, (202) 434-2277.

2. J.F. Fries, MD. *Aging Well*, Reading, MA: Addison-Wesley, 1989.

3. D.E. Larson, MD, ed. *Mayo Clinic Family Health Book*, New York, NY: William Morrow and Co., Inc., 1990.

4. Planetree Health Resource Center, 2040 Webster Street, San Francisco, CA 94115, (415) 923-3680. Planetree can prepare and mail "In-depth Research Packets" on the medical topic of your choice.

5. *Self-Care Catalog*. Call (800) 345-3371.

6. D. Vickery , MD and J.F. Fries, MD. *Take Care of Yourself* (4th Edition), Reading, MA: Addison-Wesley, 1989.

7. R.J. Weiss, MD and G. Subak-Sharpe. *Complete Guide to Health and Well-Being After 50*, New York, NY: Columbia University School of Public Health, Random House, 1988.

C. Alcohol Problems

1. *Alcoholics Anonymous: The Story of How Thousands of Men and Women Have Recovered from Alcoholism* (3rd Edition), New York, NY: Alcoholics Anonymous World Services, Inc., 1976.

2. *The Twelve Steps of Alcoholics Anonymous (Interpreted by The Hazelden Foundation)*, New York, NY: Harper and Row, 1987.

D. Alzheimer's Disease/Dementia

1. N. L. Mace and P. V. Rabins, MD. *The 36-Hour Day: A Family Guide to Caring for Persons with Alzheimer's Disease, Related Dementing Illnesses, and Memory Loss in Late Life*, Baltimore, MD: The Johns Hopkins University Press, 1991.

2. F.H. McDowell, ed. *Managing the Person with Intellectual Loss at Home*, White Plains, NY: Burke Rehabilitation Center, 1980.

(These two books are also available from the Alzheimer's Association, (800) 272-3900.)

E. Anger

1. A. Ellis. *Anger,* New York, NY: Carol Publishing Group, 1985.

2. H. Lerner. *The Dance of Anger*, New York, NY: Harper Row, 1989.

F. Anxiety

1. A. Seagrave and F. Covington. *Free From Fears*, New York, NY: Simon and Schuster, Poseidon Press, 1988.

2. C. Weeks. *More Help for Your Nerves*, New York, NY: Bantam Books, 1984.

G. Arthritis

1. K. Lorig and J.F. Fries, MD. *The Arthritis Helpbook*. Reading, MA: Addison-Wesley, 1990.

H. Assistive Devices

1. A.I. Abrams and M.A. Abrams. *The First Whole Rehab Catalog: A Comprehensive Guide to Products and Services for the Physically Disadvantaged*, White Hall, VA: Betterway Publications, Inc., 1990.

I. Asthma

1. The American Lung Association, 1991. "*Help Yourself to Better Breathing*," available from your local chapter of the American Lung Association.

2. A. Weinstein, MD. *Asthma: The Complete Guide to Self-Management of Asthma for Patients and Their Families*, New York, NY: McGraw-Hill, 1987.

J. Caregiving

1. "*How to Hire Helpers: A Guide for Elders and Their Families*," The Church Council of Greater Seattle, 4759 15th Street, NW, Seattle, WA 98105.

2. "*Miles Away and Still Caring: A Guide for Long-Distance Caregivers*," 1987. Available from the American Association of Retired Persons, 601 E Street, NW, Washington, DC 20049, (202) 434-2277.

K. Depression

1. D. Burns, MD. *The Feeling Good Handbook*, New York, NY: New American Library, 1990.

2. M. Seligman. *Learned Optimism*, New York, NY: Random House, 1991.

L. Diabetes

1. L. Jovanovic-Peterson, MD, C.M. Peterson, MD, and M.B. Stone. *A Touch of Diabetes--A Guide for People Who Have Type II, Non-Insulin Dependent Diabetes*, Minneapolis, MN: DCI Publishing, 1991.

M. Fitness

1. D. Chrisman. *Body Recall*, (5th Edition), Dorothy Chrisman, P.O. Box 363, Berea College, Berea, KY 40404, (606) 986-2181.

2. *Pep up Your Life: A Fitness Book for Seniors*, 1987. Available from the American Association of Retired Persons, 601 E Street, NW, Washington, DC 20049, (202) 434-2277.

N. Grief

1. E. Neeld. *Seven Choices*. New York, NY: Crown, 1990.

2. H.S. Schiff. *Living Through Mourning: Finding Comfort and Hope When a Loved One Has Died*, New York, NY: Penguin Books, 1986.

O. Incontinence

1. K.L. Burgis, MD, K.L Pearce, and A.L. Lucco, MD. *Staying Dry: A Practical Guide to Bladder Control*, Baltimore, MD: The Johns Hopkins University Press, 1989.

2. C.B. Gartley. *Managing Incontinence*, 1985. Available from the Simon Foundation, P.O. Box 835, Wilmette, IL, 60091, (800) 237-4666.

P. Medical Consumerism

1. C. Inlander and E. Weiner. *Take This Book to the Hospital With You*, Emmaus, PA: Rodale Press, 1985.

2. D.R. Stutz, MD and B. Feder. *The Savvy Patient: How to be an Active Participant in Your Medical Care*, Mt. Vernon, NY: Consumers Union, 1990.

3. U.S. Department of Health and Human Services, Health Care Financing Administration. *The Medicare 1991 Handbook*, available from your local Social Security Administration office or from HCFA, 6325 Security Blvd., Baltimore, MD 21207.

Q. Medications

1. J. Graedon and T. Graedon. *50+: The Graedon's People's Pharmacy for Older Adults*, available from Graedon Enterprises, Inc., P.O. Box 52027, Durham, NC 27717-2027.

2. J.W. Long, MD. *The Essential Guide to Prescription Drugs, 1992: Everything You Need to Know for Safe Drug Use*, New York, NY: HarperCollins Publishers, 1992.

3. *Physician's Desk Reference*. Available at most hospital and public libraries.

R. Memory

1. K.B. Gose and G.H. Levi. *Dealing with Memory Changes as You Grow Older,* 1985. This book can be ordered from Gloria Levi, 3856 West 12th Avenue, Vancouver, British Columbia, CANADA V6R 2N8.

S. Mental Self-Care/Mental Wellness

1. G. Emery and J. Campbell. *Rapid Relief from Emotional Distress*, New York, NY: Rawson Associates, 1986.

2. D.W. Kemper, *et al. Growing Wiser: The Older Person's Guide to Mental Wellness,* Healthwise, Inc., 1986. Available from Healthwise, P.O. Box 1989, Boise, ID 83701.

3. S. Locke, MD and D. Colligan. *The Healer Within*, New York, NY: New American Library, 1986.

4. R. Ornstein and D. Sobel, MD. *The Healing Brain*, New York, NY: Simon and Schuster, 1987.

T. Newsletters

1. *Consumer Reports Health Letter*, P.O. Box 56356, Boulder, CO 80322-6356.

2. *The Johns Hopkins Medical Letter: Health After 50*, P.O. Box 420179, Palm Coast, FL 32142.

3. *University of California at Berkeley Wellness Letter*, P.O. Box 420148, Palm Coast, FL 32142.

U. Pain

1. E.M. Catalan. *The Chronic Pain Workbook: A Step-by-Step Guide for Coping with and Overcoming Your Pain*, Oakland, CA: New Harbinger Publications, 1987.

V. Safety

1. American Association of Retired Persons "*55 Alive/Mature Driving*" Course. Contact your local AARP office for information.

2. American Automobile Association Foundation for Traffic Safety, 1730 M Street, NW, Suite 401, Washington, DC 20036, (202) 775-1456.

3. Consumer Product Safety Commission publication, "*Safety for Older Consumers Home Safety Checklist*," January, 1985. Consumer Product Safety Commission. (800) 638-2772.

W. Smoking

1. T. Ferguson, MD. *The No-Nag, No-Guilt, Do-It-Your-Own-Way Guide to Quitting Smoking*, New York, NY: Ballantine Books, 1987.

X. Stress

1. H. Benson, MD and M. Klipper. *The Relaxation Response*, New York, NY: Avon Books, 1976.

Y. Women's Health

1. P.B. Doress and D.L. Siegal. *Ourselves, Growing Older*, New York, NY: Simon and Schuster, 1987.

2. M. Feltin. *A Woman's Guide to Good Health After 50.* Greenville, IL: Scott, Foresman, and Company, 1987. Available from AARP Books/Scott, Foresman, and Company, 1865 Miner Street, Des Plaines, IL 60057-0702.

MEDICATIONS INDEX

The following prescription, over-the-counter, and generic medications are mentioned in the text. Brand names are included as examples only. Mention of a particular product or brand does not imply an endorsement of that product.

A

Acetaminophen, **336**
Advil, 145, 337
Aldoclor, 145
Aldomet, 145
Aldoril, 145
Alka-2, 331
Alka-Seltzer, 331
Alpha-Keri, 187
Alprazolam, 145
Alzapam, 145
Amitril, 145
Amitriptyline, 145
Amoxicillin, 338
Amphojel, 331
Ampicillin, 338
Anaprox, 145
Antacids, **331**
Antibiotics, 212, **337**
Anticholinergics, 145
Anticoagulants, 184
Antidepressants, 103, 145, 146, 223, 333, 335
Anti-diarrheals, **332**
Antihistamines, 87, 108, 145, 223, **333**
Antihypertensives, 145, 146, 219
Aspirin, 107, 111, **336**
Ativan, 145, 245
Atropine, 145
Augmentin, 338

B

Bacitracin, 346
Bactrim, 338
Balneol, 109

Ben-Gay, 66
Benadryl, 170, 187, 333
Bentyl, 145
Benzocaine, 177
Blistex, 171
Bromo Seltzer, 331
Burrow's solution, 187

C

Campho-Phenique, 171
Catapres, 145
Ceclor, 338
Cefaclor, 338
Cephradine, 338
Cefadroxil, 338
Cephalexin, 338
Chlor-Trimeton, 187, 333, 346
Chlordiazepoxide, 145
Chlorpheniramine, 333
Chlorpromazine, 145
Cimetidine, 145
CIPRO, 338
Clonidine, 145
Coricidin, 333
Codeine, 145, 245
Correctol, 336
Cortaid, 346

D

Dalmane, 245, 339
Darvon, 245
Decongestants, 87, **334**
Demerol, 245
Demi-Regroton, 145
Desenex, 188
Dextromethorphan, 335
Di-Gel, 332
Diazepam, 145
Diclonine hydrochloride, 177
Dicloxacillin, 338
Dicyclomine, 145
Digoxin, 145

N

Naprosyn, 111, 145
Naproxen, 111, 145
Nembutal, 245
Neo-synephrine, 334
Nitrofurantoin, 338
Nuprin, 145, 337

O

Orabase, 170
Oreticyl, 145

P

Parkinson's drugs, 145
Parepectolin, 332
Penicillin G, 338
Penicillin VK, 338
Pentazine, 145
Percodan, 245
Petroleum jelly, 187, 346
Phenergan, 145
Phenobarbital, 245
Phenylephrine, 334
Phenytoin, 145
Phillip's Milk of Magnesia, 331
Promapar, 145
Promethazine, 145
Propanolol, 145
Prorex, 145
Pseudoephedrine, 334

R

Ranitidine, 145
Rauzide, 145
Regroton, 145
Reserpine, 145
Restoril, 339
Riopan, 332
Robitussin, 335, 346
Robitussin-AC, 145
Robitussin-DM, 335, 346

S

Seconal, 245

Septra, 338
Ser-Ap-Es, 145
Serpalan, 145
Sinemet, 145
Sleeping pills, 145, 252, **339**
Sonazine, 145
Spec-T, 177
Sucrets Maximum Strength, 177
Sudafed, 334
Surgilube, 210
Syntex, 187

T

Tagamet, 145
Tetracycline, 338
Thorazine, 145
Tinactin, 188
Tofranil, 145
Tranquilizers, 145, 223, 333, **339**
Tranxene, 339
Triaminic, 333
Triavil, 145
Tucks, 109
TUMS, 50, 331, 346
Tylenol, 336
Tylenol-3, 145
Tyrobenz, 177

U

Unipres, 145

V

Valium, 145, 245, 339
Valrelease, 145
Vaseline, 108, 187, 346
Vazepam, 145
Vicks VapoRub, 66

X

Xanax, 145, 339
Xerolube, 175

Z

Zantac, 145
Zinc oxide, 108

GENERAL INDEX

M